When Autumn Leaves Start to Fall

Living with Lewy Body Dementia

By Teddie Potter

When Autumn Leaves Start to Fall
Living with Lewy Body Dementia

ISBN: 978-1-7371445-5-7

Publisher: Destiny Publishings'
Editing: Cynthia Valentine
Cover Design: Safeer Ahmed

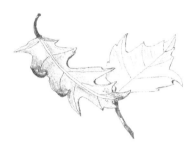

Dedication

This book is dedicated to my fantastic extended family who loved, supported, and helped me through this heartbreaking journey. I don't know what I would have done without them!

Many thanks to author and nurse, Gail Weatherhill for her informative and inspiring book, "The Caregiver's Guide to Dementia." These words from her introduction touched my core.

"Hold tight to the person your loved one still is. And never doubt that what the brain cannot remember, the heart cannot forget."

Introduction

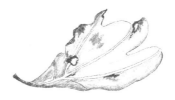

Autumn leaves drift down
Tossed away by the cold wind
Like his thoughts, scattered

The lovely song, "Autumn Leaves", by Johnny Mercer ends "But I miss you most of all, my darling, when autumn leaves start to fall." Those words always invoked a feeling of melancholy: the end of summer, the forecast of a cold, long winter. But when my husband developed Lewy Body dementia, they meant even more. The falling leaves symbolized the slow shedding of his memories, his reason, his health – and finally his life.

Preface

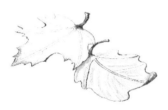

Quality of Life?
Remember every teardrop
Treasure each smile

When my husband, Don, was diagnosed with unspecified dementia in 2018, I was angry, scared, and totally unprepared. As the disease progressed, I always felt that I was one step behind. I didn't know the right questions to ask and didn't anticipate the next crisis. Then, all the books I read were about Alzheimer's disease and barely mentioned the hallucinations, delusions, and intense acting-out dreams characteristic of Lewy Body dementia (LBD).

I have a doctorate in educational leadership which helped me do research but didn't equip me to deal with this dreaded disease. I'm not a qualified doctor, lawyer, or financial advisor, so I cannot give professional advice in those fields. However, I can relate my own personal experiences and what I learned along this journey. Everyone is different and LBD does not progress in a predictable and linear way. So do your own research (resources are listed at the end of this book) and consult with your family and your own advisors.

I have divided the chapters into two sections. The first part is the story of our battle with Lewy Body dementia. The second section is a list of things that I learned – and wished I had known earlier. For convenience I have used the pronouns he, him and his. Please note that while men tend to develop LBD more often than women, anyone can develop this dreaded disease. In these pages, I explain what worked and didn't work for me and my loved one (LO). Please use what you can.

I have included my little haikus, watercolor paintings and ink sketches because creating them during the seven years we struggled with LBD helped keep me sane. The autumn leaves deteriorate and wither, symbolizing the devastation that LBD causes to its victims. And winter always comes.

Living with LBD is a long, hard road. Try to savor the moments of joy and cling to the good memories. I sincerely hope this book helps you cope with this heartbreaking disease. God bless.

Table of Contents

Green Leaves.. 1

Summer Leaves 11

Autumn Leaves... 19

Brown Leaves.. 34

Withered Leaves.. 58

Winter Leaves 84

Green Leaves

Green leaves of summer
Vibrant and healthy
Full of promise and hope

Like the green leaves of summer, Don and I felt healthy and full of vitality. We looked forward to our old age, anticipating many more years of enjoying each other, our friends and family, and contributing to our community. We had never heard of Lewy Body Dementia.

Don proposed to me while ghost-hunting the Maco Light in North Carolina. Neither of us was ready for marriage. I had finished my first year of college and was saving for a backpacking trip through Europe. He had been commissioned to First Lieutenant in the Marine Corps and was looking for adventure. We spent a summer exploring the beaches of North Carolina, searching for the perfect hush puppy in his little Marine Corps green sports car. It convinced us that we did not want to lose each other!

I was a Marine Corps brat, so I knew what I was getting into. We had a lovely wedding in the chapel on Camp Lejeune, with a reception at the Officer's Club and an open bar (a time-honored tradition in the Marine Corps!). A month later, Don was deployed aboard a warship blockading Cuba during the Cuban Missile Crisis! Welcome to the life of a Marine Corps wife. The old saying goes, "If the Corps had wanted you to have a wife and family, they would have issued you one!". God, country, corps, and then family have always been the priorities of a Marine.

Nevertheless, we did manage to have a family: three beautiful, intelligent, and very active boys. Greg was born while Don was stationed at the National Security Agency, and Don didn't see him until he was three days old. He was home for Brad, born fifteen months later – a lucky coincidence. The youngest, David, was born when Don was serving his first tour in Vietnam.

I met Don in San Francisco when he returned. (Leaving all three boys -aged three years, eighteen months, and six months - with my supportive and soon-to-be exhausted parents.) Don and I had a marvelous time exploring that beautiful city. One day we wandered down to the Haight Ashbury district. We strolled through the streets, full of colorful hippies, a haze of pot, and protest music. Even in civilian clothes, Don looked like a Marine, crewcut, clean-shaven, straight, and tall. A little whisp of a girl approached him and handed him a flower. "Make love, not war.", she intoned. Don replied, "I intend to, ma'am."

I didn't get my tour of Europe until we retired, but Don definitely got his share of adventure: two tours in Vietnam, jungle warfare school, aerial observation training in Norway, winter warfare school, desert combat training, three years as head of the Marine security detail at the embassy in Germany, and countless deployments for maneuvers in the Caribbean. One winter, he was sent to New York with an air squadron. During an unexpected winter blizzard, he and his crew were snowed in for several days – in the officer's club. I was home with three boys with chicken pox!

Don had his softer side. One evening in Germany, the boys came home carrying a tiny, curly black puppy. "The neighbors gave him to us. Can we keep him PLEEESE?" Now Don was head of the US Marine Corps Embassy Security Group for the American Embassy in Bonn, West Germany. He looked at the cute little wiggling pup and sighed. "Guys, I lead the Marines. I can't have a poodle!" But he gave in, and the Marines named the dog, Chesty, after a war hero. Chesty ran five miles every morning with the Marines and then played all afternoon with the boys. He traveled all over northern Europe with us in our Volkswagen camper. Don loved him!

When the boys grew older, we would all gather for the holidays and inevitably start telling "Don stories." One of our all-time favorites was our survivor camping trip to the Outer Banks of North Carolina. Don didn't go on vacations – he went on missions. So, I was constantly inventing reasons to go to the Florida Keys – the boys wanted to learn how to scuba dive. Or, we had to go on that windjammer cruise to the Bahamas because all the boys had to write essays on "what I did on my summer vacation."

This time we told Don we needed to go to the beach on the Outer Banks because the boys needed to earn their Boy Scout survival camping badge.

It was early fall, and the beaches were almost deserted. We had arranged for a fishing boat to take us to an uninhabited island where we planned to stay for three days. We were carting in our water, MREs (meals- ready-to-eat), medical supplies, tents, matches – and of course, a KaBar Marine Corp all-purpose knife. We loaded all the supplies aboard, and Don lined us up on the wooden dock for a last-minute briefing. All three boys, Chesty, and I stood at parade rest while Don began his lecture. He reminded us that there were no phones or first aid stations on the island and that we would have to be careful and alert. "Situational awareness is essential. Always be aware of your surroundings." he intoned. And then, he accidentally stepped back and fell off the dock into the cold Atlantic water. The best part of the story came later.

A surprise hurricane threatened the Outer Banks, and on the second day, a fishing boat came to evacuate us from the island. The winds were howling, and the waves were breaking over the sides of the tiny vessel. I went first, jumping from the dock to the rocking deck of the boat. Then Don helped each boy jump over, tossed the dog to me, and leaped into the boat. We arrived safely at the fishing dock and quickly unloaded all the gear. As we thanked the ship's captain, Don saluted and stepped back off the dock into the water again. No one dared laugh. "Situational Awareness" became our code words for "Don't do anything stupid!"

After retiring from the Marines and teaching JROTC for seven years, Don decided to earn his doctorate. The boys had all finished college and started their grown-up lives, so we moved to Athens, Georgia. Don became the oldest Graduate Assistant in the history of the University. We truly enjoyed those years. I was teaching full time, and we would meet after school in Athens and sit at one of the downtown outdoor cafés, and people watch. We felt like college kids again.

I was teaching gifted middle school students, and my class decided we needed to do something hands-on. After much research, we decided to build an electric-powered go-cart. I spent that summer taking a college correspondence class on basic electrical theory, and Don worked with an electrical engineer to create plans to build "Panther's Speed." That middle school course became a statewide competition. Trophies were given for scientific knowledge, driving, troubleshooting, and an informational skit. I was paid to teach the class, attend seminars and workshops, and the electrical vehicle rallies. Don volunteered to show the students how to build the cart, troubleshoot, and drive it safely. We won the State Championship twice! My principal later wrote that Don was "not just a volunteer, but a philanthropist, generously giving his time, expertise, and enthusiasm to help educate our students."

We built our dream house when Don got a job teaching at Piedmont College. It was big enough for all the grandkids to visit, a bike ride away from the lake and our kayaks, and three and a half acres of woods and gardens to explore. Don bought a little Cessna airplane and started a small aerial photography business. We both were avid community volunteers and travelers. We explored other countries and enjoyed whitewater rafting, hang gliding, and horseback riding. For our 50th wedding anniversary, we went to Greece. We climbed the stairs to the Parthenon, swam in the Aegean, rode horses in the hills over Naxos harbor, and watched the sunset in Santorini. However, our lives were about to change.

What I Learned:

1. Dementia is not a disease, but a condition caused by many medical problems that usually surface when the brain is injured. It is defined as a disorder that manifests as related symptoms that typically appear when the brain is damaged due to trauma or disease. The symptoms involve progressive impairments in memory, thinking, and behaviors, significantly impacting an individual's ability to deal with all facets of everyday living. In the USA, over 6 million people over 65 are diagnosed with some form of dementia each year. The odds of someone you know and love contracting dementia are very likely.

Alzheimer's is a neurodegenerative disease that usually starts slowly and progressively worsens. Approximately 60-70% of cases of dementia are the result of Alzheimer's disease. It is characterized by short-term memory loss, problems with language, disorientation, mood swings, and behavioral issues. The causes are poorly understood, and no effective treatment or cure exists.

Vascular dementia results from a decreased flow of blood to the brain. A progressive decline in thinking skills is the main symptom. It can be mitigated by treating the cause of vascular problems.

Creutzfeldt-Jakob disease, also known as "mad cow" disease, is caused by virus-like particles called prions. It is usually caused by contaminated meat or infected medical equipment. It progresses rapidly, and there is no effective treatment or cure.

Frontotemporal dementia, or Prick's disease, attacks the frontal and temporal lobes of the brain. It causes drastic personality changes and loss of social skills, language problems, and, eventually, memory decline. There seems to be a genetic cause and no treatment or cure.

Parkinson's disease is a chronic degenerative nervous system disorder that mainly affects the motor system. The main symptoms are tremors, rigidity, and balance issues. However, cognitive decline and hallucinations can occur later. As there is no cure, treatment aims to reduce symptoms.

Lewy Body dementia is a degenerative brain disease that causes a progressive decline in cognitive functioning. It is the second most common kind of neurodegenerative dementia after Alzheimer's. LBD ultimately leads to the irreversible loss of intellectual and functional capacity. Patients with this disease present sleep and behavioral problems, delusions, and vivid hallucinations. Many patients experience intense, acting-out dreams. The exact cause of LBD is unknown, and the average life expectancy after diagnosis is four years.

Some symptoms of Lewy Body Dementia are evident long before mental cognition declines. Most people suffering from LBD have sleep disorders, and many have experienced vivid and intense dreams and nightmares. One night Don punched a hole in the wall next to our bed because he thought he was wrestling a python! A change in gait and balance problems are early signs. Also, the sense of smell seems to diminish in many patients.

2. While you and your LO are healthy and thinking clearly, is the time to set your medical and financial affairs in order. Obtaining the documents, you need becomes much more difficult after your LO becomes impaired. Here are some steps you should consider taking.

A will may be needed to list what will become of a LO's material possessions at their time of death. It may prevent the LO's estate from going before a probate judge who could divide assets equally between closest relatives. A will may also avert family disputes about who gets grandma's antique piano or that valuable stamp collection.

An advanced directive for health care or a living will is a legal document designed to state the LO's directives regarding his future health care and to assist the designated health agent act when a LO cannot make his own decisions. It will state the individual's preferences regarding prolonging or not prolonging life in such matters as using feeding tubes, CPR, or other life support systems.

A durable power of attorney is designed to give the legal authority to one person to act for another person. If a LO does become unable to make informed decisions, then the DPA allows the designated agent to sell a house or car or place the LO in an assisted living facility. This should be done BEFORE your LO is diagnosed with dementia. Both Don and I signed a durable power of attorney. He listed me as his agent. However, without his knowledge, I recorded our eldest son as my agent.

Add your name to all accounts to avoid complications when your LO is diagnosed with dementia or dies. The power of attorney is no longer recognized when a LO dies, so it's automatically frozen if you are not a co-owner of a bank account. You should also see if the bank requires a separate power of attorney.

3.   This is the time to talk with your LO about finances. Ensure you know the passwords to all bank accounts, credit cards, insurance, investment, and pension plans. Record the security questions for each account. In a few years, you may need to remember the correct answers! Keep a duplicate copy of the information in a safe place. I never knew that Don had a monthly allotment to the Navy Federal Credit Union or that he had purchased accidental death protection when he bought his airplane.

Sometimes your loved LO doesn't want to discuss financial and legal matters. "We're healthy. We have plenty of time." "Don't worry about finances. We're fine." I appealed to Don's sense of organization and said it was always better to be prepared. Fortunately, one of our sons is a lawyer, so he was able to bring over some forms and make an appointment with a friend who specialized in wills. I also made an appointment with our CPA on the pretense that we needed to ensure we understood all of the tax implications for using Don's airplane in an aerial photography business. I made out a long list of other questions to ask.

Talk to an estate planner and see what the rules are in your state. Medicare doesn't pay for assisted living, memory care, nursing homes, or nursing home care. Medicaid can only be used when you've exhausted all your other resources, and it has stringent rules about giving away your money or home to your children. We found out too late that Georgia has a plan where the spouse of a person in a care facility can separate her income and set up a trust for the spouse's money. That way, only the assets in the LO's name are counted toward the Medicaid threshold. It's worth the rather steep lawyer's fee to see if there is a way to help you save money in the future.

.

Summer Leaves

Struggling with laces
Fumbling with buttons
I watch him, and cry inside

The leaves of summer change so slowly that we often don't realize they are dying. I knew something was wrong but didn't know precisely what was happening.

It started with the shuffling. Don went from running three miles every other day to dragging his feet and hunching his back. He fell down the back stairs and needed stitches after tripping in the backyard. Our conversations became a litany of "Honey, I can't find my phone!"…wallet, pen, keys, etc. Our credit score decreased because he forgot to pay the bills, and his photographs were out of focus. At first, I tried to compensate. I put up grab bars and a railing in the backyard. I placed a bright red bowl on the entry table and reminded him to put his things there. I convinced him it would be easier to put all the bills on the computer and pay them automatically. I even photoshopped his pictures. I was more annoyed than concerned. Everyone gets older and more absentminded, I told myself. "No real problem."

In 2015, Don hurt his back. He was working at the Lion's Club annual car show and tossed a heavy box into a pickup truck. The next day he couldn't get out of bed. We went to our primary doctor, who pronounced it a strained muscle, and gave him some pain medicine -oxycodone. The pain just got worse. We went to the orthopedic clinic, and they took X-rays, which showed that he had a compressed disk fracture. They gave him a muscle relaxer and more oxycodone. Don couldn't sleep or walk because he was in such severe pain. Then his pain seemed to move. Given his history of kidney stones, we went to our urologist. We discovered he had two kidney stones.

The urologist used a laser to pulverize them. After the procedure, they prescribed bed rest and more pain meds. Don was exhausted, confused, and depressed. He slept in his recliner in his basement study, and I climbed stairs all day, delivering food, meds, and comfort.

A month later, Don woke up in the middle of the night, unable to urinate and in even more pain. I couldn't imagine what was wrong. I called my pharmacist friend, who came over and talked to Don. Herschel said that he thought it was urinary retention. This is a potentially very serious condition in which a person cannot urinate. We called 911, and Emergency Medical Technicians (EMTs) carried Don upstairs from the basement. Then he was rushed to the emergency room. The urologist on call performed an emergency surgical dilation of the urethral. The doctor found Don had scar tissue growth from radiation treatments he'd received for prostate cancer years prior. The urologist put in a temporary catheter and attached a bag for the urine. So now, Don had a compressed disk fracture and a catheter bag. He was still in pain and more and more confused and forgetful. Adding to the list of complications, he developed inflammatory colitis and had to have a colonoscopy! To top off the year, he spent Christmas in bed with bronchitis, and we had to cancel our New Year plans. Both of us were exhausted.

Eventually, Don's back improved. The catheter was removed. However, he was still very forgetful and muddled. Don couldn't find the right words and tripped over the rug or the stairs. He told me that he felt like he was falling apart and was angry that the doctors couldn't seem to help. "What did I do to cause all this?"

One morning, after walking the dog, bringing Don his breakfast, putting in a load of laundry, and penciling in appointments on the big calendar I had set up in the kitchen, I sat down to drink a cup of coffee. Staring out the windows, seeing the overgrown garden, the neglected lawn, and the broken bird feeder overwhelmed me. I began crying endlessly and couldn't stop. I never wanted to be a nurse, and no matter how hard I tried, Don was still miserable.

I'm a list maker, so I started jotting down our current problems. Don had multiple medical issues and was showing signs of mental decline. He was forgetful, lost things, couldn't find the right words, and seemed addled. His balance was poor, and he fell often. His small motor coordination was also affected. He knocked over glasses, dropped things, and could no longer type on the computer. He was bored, depressed, and angry because he couldn't do what he loved – fly his airplane, go to the gym, run with the dog, or help at community events.

One evening after a glass of wine and a PBS special, Don said, "I feel so useless and helpless. I hate that you have to do so much more work, and I can't help."

All I could do was hug him and remind him of all the times he had helped me. I was exhausted and frightened. My description of myself had always been "I am an optimistic pessimist." Through all our years of married life, I knew bad things would happen, but I always felt I could cope." Now, I wasn't so sure.

I didn't know what was causing all of Don's problems. None of the doctors had an answer. We had seen several specialists, and they found no problems except the pain in Don's back and mild high blood pressure. My back and knee were causing me more and more pain as I tried to keep up with all the chores and take care of Don. I decided to do my own research, get some household help and hire a yard man. We weren't traveling anymore, so we had some extra money. Armed with a plan, I went downstairs to bring Don his clean laundry.

He was sitting on the commode, hunched over and shaking. I went in and hugged him. "What's wrong? How can I help?" Don replied," I can't have a BM, and my back and stomach hurt." He had been very constipated since the doctors started him on oxycodone. We tried prune juice, laxatives, and more water. Nothing seemed to work. However, this was the first time he could not have a bowel movement. I called his urologist, and the doctor told me to take Don to the emergency room.

I called my neighbor and asked her to check on the dog, threw some extra clothes and his meds into the car, and we took off. It was a Friday afternoon, so the ER in Athens, Georgia, was relatively empty. Don was shivering, moaning, and rocking back and forth. We checked in and were informed that there had been a wreck on Highway 441, and all the doctors were busy. We waited over an hour. Don and I were in tears when the nurse took us back to a room.

The room was small, cold, and furnished with a small bed, a tiny table, and a straight-backed chair. Don was undressed on the bed and covered with a hospital gown and a light blanket. The doctor finally came in and asked me what was going on. Don was unable to talk coherently, so I explained. The doctor glared at me and said, "Didn't you know that oxycodone causes severe constipation? Why did you let him get in this state?"

They tried to give Don an enema. When that didn't work, they gave him a mild sedative to relax him. Then the doctor put on gloves, spread cream on Don's rectum, and inserted his finger. He dug out big, dried hunks of feces while the nurse held Don down, and I cried. That night I slept on the sofa in the study so I could help Don go to the bathroom – all night long.

The next day I sent my sister and three sons a long text describing what was happening and asking for help. I knew I could no longer cope by myself. I started searching the web for answers and hired a housekeeper. I resigned as president of the local arts council and started looking for a smaller, safer house. Our golden years were beginning to tarnish.

What I Learned:

1. Dementia may be triggered or worsen when a LO has a physical problem or trauma. Some doctors even recommend not having elective surgery if it means going under anesthesia. Almost all medications have side effects and can cause constipation. Oxycodone often causes confusion and severe constipation. Research the medications prescribed, and don't be afraid to ask your doctor questions. Keep a journal of what medications your LO is taking and the effect on his symptoms and overall health.

2. As many different conditions can cause dementia, you should convince your LO to visit various specialists to rule out vascular dementia, a brain tumor, or some other cause. However, specialists are sometimes like blind men and the elephant. They only focus on one part of the whole. It's up to you as a caregiver to keep good notes and ask questions. "What are the side effects of this medication? Will it interfere with the medications he is already taking?" You must be your LO's advocate. Start a journal of his symptoms, medications, operations, and procedures that he has had.

I asked Don's doctors and everyone we did business with to call or email me instead of Don. He often forgot to tell me about appointments or essential information.

3. After one of Don's many trips to the emergency room for falls, urinary retention, and impacted bowels, he was admitted for the night. I found out that this triggered a series of visits by Medicare nurses. We had a nurse come to evaluate Don, and she recommended physical therapy, occupational therapy, and a short mental screening. The team came for six weeks, helped Don with exercises, and showed me how to make our house safer. I never knew that resource was available.

4. Start doing your own research. You can find reliable information on the Dementia Association's website and other sources such as the Mayo Clinic, AARP, the National Institute of Aging, and the Lewy Body Dementia Association. (References are listed at the end of this book) Discuss what you learned with your doctor. Remember, you and your LO are the experts on his symptoms and feelings. If your doctor doesn't listen, consider changing doctors.

5. Every book, article, or website you visit will emphasize one thing: caregiving is challenging and exhausting. You need to take care of yourself and build a support network. I found myself feeling angry and sorry for myself. I was tired and stressed. Most of my time was spent caring for Don, the house, the finances, etc. Then I'd think about what Don was experiencing. I would feel so guilty! I'd blame myself for losing my temper, not doing enough to keep him comfortable, and not being a good wife.

6. Remember, you are not perfect. You can only do so much. Talk to a friend, a counselor, or a trusted advisor. Ask for assistance. When a family member or a friend asks how they can help, have a list ready! "Could you pick up the cleaning for me when you go to the grocery store? Or "Would you be able to take Don out for breakfast on Monday morning? I want to go to exercise class." When you can't handle things, step outside, recite the Serenity Prayer, and just breathe.

If you are fortunate to have a friend who will let you vent, you are truly blessed. My sister, Sandra, listened to my problems, offered advice, and gave me much-needed emotional support.

Autumn Leaves

My husband, my friend
Father of my sons
No longer the man I knew

Autumn leaves turn red and gold, disguising the little imperfections and discoloration that foretell the coming of winter. I was still blaming Don's cognitive decline on his medical problems. We both truly hoped that it was true.

Don and I sat on the patio drinking coffee and watching the hummingbirds fight over the birdfeeder and our little mutt, Recon, tenaciously trying to dig out a cunning chipmunk. I brought up the subject of downsizing. Don was absolutely against it. He had worked so hard on our yard, hauling rocks to make a dry creek bed, bushwacking a trail down to the creek, and digging holes so I could plant trees and flowers. We loved being near the lake, the walking trails, and enjoyed our neighbors.

Our house was built by a good friend who was a contractor. Don helped build the rock fireplace in the living room, and I had carefully picked out the huge windows facing our front yard. It was big enough for family Thanksgiving gatherings and neighborhood block parties. We had memorabilia from all our trips and three large boxes of Christmas tree ornaments. Neither of us wanted to leave.

Don reminded me that he had already sold his beloved "Skylark" airplane, and now I was asking him to get rid of even more precious belongings. "I feel like I'm being stripped of my identity, layer by layer."

Thanks to the magic of cellphone technology, the boys and I had been texting each other regularly while Don was watching TV. They were incredibly supportive and helpful, but all had different ideas. Don and I could move in with one of the boys, try an assisted living facility, or get a condo by the beach. I gradually introduced Don to all those ideas, and we decided to start looking at options. Don kept saying he would be fine as soon as he could return to the gym. However, we both knew that things would not get any better.

One of our first ideas was moving into a smaller house near the beach. We took short vacations exploring the Golden Isles in Georgia and the coast of Florida. It gave us both something to do, but we quickly realized we couldn't be far away from family and friends. Don couldn't go for more than an hour or two without looking for a bathroom. Often our road trips were canceled because of his alternating bouts of diarrhea and constipation. And I realized that even with GPS, Don couldn't find his way around. More and more, he let me drive.

So, we went with our eldest son, Greg, to look at a continuous care community nearby. It was beautiful: lovely grounds, saltwater inside the swimming pool, several different dining options, and a cornucopia of activities. The idea was that residents paid a one-time entrance fee and then could move into a small apartment on the grounds. As we aged and required more services, those could be added at no extra charge. There was even a memory care unit on the grounds. We had a lovely lunch at the facility and toured the kayaks on the lake. Then we sat down with the admission agent. The upfront buy-in cost was about $300,000 plus a monthly fee of about $6000. I smiled sweetly, said we were still weighing our options and appreciated the tour and information. Once back at our car, Greg and I couldn't stop laughing. If we had that much money, we'd hire a maid, gardener, and full-time nurse!

Most assisted living quarters were tiny and depressing, so we looked at "over-fifty" communities. These seemed ideal. Most communities had smaller, one-story homes with safety features like grab bars in the bathrooms and doors wide enough for wheelchairs. Usually, they had clubhouses and recreation facilities. Often lawn care is covered by the Homeowner's Association fee. The problem was that there were very few in our area available. Whenever a home went on the market, it was snapped up immediately.

Nevertheless, we put our home on the market. I must admit I enjoyed "staging" it. We had it inspected and assessed. We fixed the front door entranceway, cleaned the rugs, hired a gardener, and manicured the yard. It looked so great that I lay awake nights trying to figure out ways to stay. Could we install mechanical seats that took you up and down staircases? Find someone willing to be a live-in maid for room and board and a small salary.

Then Don would trip coming in from the garage, or I would twist my knee going upstairs, and reality would prevail. As much as we hated the thought, we knew we had to find some-place smaller and safer.

So, the hard part began -downsizing. Don declared that he wouldn't give the small gauge train set he purchased in Germany to just anyone. We had to find someone who would really appreciate it. I hated the thought of giving away the Christmas ornaments we had brought back from overseas, the ones given to me by my students and especially the ones that the boys had made over the years. My sister had to come and sit beside me as I went through all three big boxes. She would pick up an ornament and ask, "What's the story behind this one?" If I couldn't come up with a touching tale, she would toss it into a box for Habitat for Humanity or someone in the family.

Don agonized over his "stuff." Fortunately, we had hired a fantastic young woman to help, and she finally put out four big boxes in the basement labeled THROW AWAY, GIVE AWAY, DONATE, KEEP. She played some of Don's favorite country music and tackled his workroom. She soon had him laughing and helping her decide which one of the four hammers he should keep.

It was helpful that we had this task because taking Don out was becoming harder and harder. When we went to the Lions Club's meetings, he would talk too loud, jump up to take a picture (even though he couldn't operate the camera anymore.), or spill his drink on the floor. I took him to a JROTC county field day and left him sitting on the bleachers while I went to park the car. When I came back, I couldn't find him. It took several JROTC instructors and multiple students to search the area and locate him. Don was tired, thirsty, confused, and in pain from his back. He told me he thought one of the high schools might need him to judge an event.

The constant coming and going of maintenance specialists, realtors, and folks helping me pack stimulated Don. People would poke their heads into the study and see all of Don's medals and awards. They always made some comments and thanked Don for his military service. That really cheered him up. Now and then, I'd see glimpses of the old Don. We had some flying squirrels removed from our attic. One night, we kept hearing scratching and mewing sounds. Armed with a fly swatter and bug spray, I climbed into the attic and saw a pitiful little flying squirrel caught in a sticky trap the rodent remover guy had left. The poor baby was in bad shape. Don took him, washed his feet, and clipped his fur so we could unglue him. Then for a week, he fed the squirrel from an eye dropper. Once it was moving around, we let it go into the forest.

We finally sold the house but didn't have a place to stay! Fortunately, a friend of a friend agreed to rent us a tiny house he was renovating on a month-to-month basis. Again, family and friends helped us pack boxes, decide what to put in storage and what we had to take. We moved into this little cottage with a small front porch and a tin roof. We stacked boxes of clothes, meds, a coffee pot, and the file cabinet in the second bedroom. We used folding tables and chairs for the TV, printer, and computer. The neighborhood was delightful, just outside of Athens. It was an eclectic mix of retirees, young families, and college students. You could walk to a local café, and the community had local bands and singers perform every second Saturday. We could walk the dog to the park and sit on the porch in the evenings. Don's back was healing, and he was less uptight and confused. I was very hopeful.

A good friend called me one evening and told me that a neighbor had just died, and his house was going up for sale. I immediately called our realtor, and we made an appointment to see it. It was in an over fifty community of eighty houses, only about ten miles from our old home. It was small but had space for Don's office and a tiny workshop/guest bedroom for me.

Don loved that the backyard opened onto the retaining pond and a forest. We bought it the next day.

The neighborhood seemed perfect: friendly people, a clubhouse with a small swimming pool, sidewalks, and a lot of trees – we loved it. We fenced in the backyard, and I started a garden. Don could walk the dog and stop and chat with other pet owners. However, his symptoms slowly began to change and worsen. "Teddie, why are all these cats in the house?"

I didn't know what to say. There were no cats in the house. Don started having more and more hallucinations. I searched the internet looking for information. It seemed that some dementia patients did hallucinate, but experts seemed to disagree with how to handle them. Reality therapy proponents state that the caregiver should gently say, "Honey, there are no cats in the house." Other experts suggested that you ask your LO to describe what he saw and distract them. If he asked if you saw it, tell him the truth. Don was very reluctant to accept that there was anything wrong with him, but he couldn't ignore the hallucinations.

One day while Don was napping in the recliner, I went out to walk the dog. When I returned, Don stood in the living room staring at the sofa. He turned to me and said, "They won't leave."

"Who won't leave?"

"The old men on the sofa and in my recliner. I asked them if they wanted coffee, but they won't speak."

Blinking tears, I quietly replied, "Can you describe them?"

"They're just old men with grey beards. But they won't leave! Do you see them?"

"No, Hon, I don't see them."

He walked over to me and hugged me. "You're substantial." Then he reached down and petted the dog. "Recon is substantial."

Moving to the sofa, he reached out his hand and touched where he thought the old men sat. "They aren't substantial."

"Teddie, what's happening?"

Don had always been very analytical, so I told him what I had read. We discussed what he thought he saw – children playing in his bedroom, people walking in the backyard at night, and some of our old pets curled up on the sofa. I asked if they frightened him, and he said, "No, but it is confusing not knowing what was real." He turned to me and took my hand. "Will you tell me what's real?"

"Always, I will always tell you what's real."

As the year went on, we had good times interspersed with troubling ones. We enjoyed the pool parties and bingo night. I joined the social committee, and Don liked the exercise class. But, his judgment and mental abilities continued to decline. We decided to sell his big truck, which wouldn't fit in our garage with the new Subaru. Don agreed that we didn't need two cars and drove into town to sell the truck. That afternoon I got a frantic call from Don. He was at the Miata repair place. He was almost crying, and I could barely understand his words. All I understood was he needed me immediately and gave me the address. I broke the speed limit getting there and found him in the parking lot sitting on the hood of a black, ragtop Miata sports car. He grabbed me and said, "Thank God you're here. Now it will be alright."

He had gone into the car lot to sell his truck and instead traded it for a used Miata. Then as he left the lot and pulled into traffic, he was hit by a minivan! The police declared that both drivers were at fault and told Don to drive to the Miata repair shop so he could get the headlights, front bumper, and door fixed. Don got there, got out of the car, and dropped his keys. He couldn't find them and just panicked and called me. I felt like raging at him. "Why the hell didn't you just sell the truck?"

But instead, I hugged him and found the keys. We left the car there to be fixed and went to lunch.
Another symptom confused me. Don could look right at a familiar object like a cell phone; if it were on its side or obstructed by a piece of paper, he wouldn't recognize it. He would open the refrigerator looking for a Coke and call me. "Teddie, are we out of Coke? When I went in to see, I'd found the Coke can partially obstructed by a Tupperware container. His spatial perception seemed to be diminishing. None of my readings about Alzheimer's mentioned anything like that!

I drove him to our favorite breakfast place one morning, looking forward to a good omelet and hot coffee. The parking lot was on a slight incline, and as Don climbed out of the car, he tripped. His Marine training clicked in. He rolled into a ball and did a parachute landing fall, coming to rest against another parked car. I was still struggling to get out of the car when people exploded from everywhere! Two men jumped out of their vehicle to assist, a waiter from the restaurant came running out, and a young lady said she was a nurse and knelt to help. Don didn't seem to have any broken bones or cuts, so the good Samaritans just helped him inside. Don was embarrassed and became annoyed. "Thank you, but I'm fine. No, don't call the ER." When the manager rushed up to apologize for the rough parking lot, Don said it was his fault, and he just wanted breakfast.

I profusely thanked everyone and assured the nurse that I would watch him for signs of a concussion. The restaurant didn't charge us for the meal, so I left a generous tip! Falls, loss of balance, and dragging his feet became commonplace.

Don also started sleeping more and more during the day. He would then wake up several times a night. Wandering became a problem. One night I woke up, and he wasn't in bed. I couldn't find him, so I went outside and told Recon, "Find Don!" The dog led me to the backyard, and I found Don in his underwear,

trying to climb in a window! He thought he heard a noise and
went out to check on it. But he locked the door and couldn't get
back in. So, I changed the door alarm code and didn't tell him.
Later, I discovered that this phenomenon is called "sundowning" and is a frequent symptom of dementia.

Nightmares became more and more frequent. Don would
wake up yelling that the house was on fire and we had to escape.
He dreamed he was a little boy back on the farm and urinated
into the trashcan, thinking it was the outhouse. Early one morning, he threw himself out of bed and wedged himself between
the bed and the wall. I couldn't move him, but I managed to
wedge a stool under his bottom. He said his back was broken,
and not knowing what else to do, I called 911.

The two young men who arrived looked like linebackers
for the UGA Bulldogs. One stepped over Don and lifted him so
the other could grab him and put him back on the bed. Don was
still complaining that his back hurt, so the guys put him on a
stretcher and took off for the hospital. I put the house key under
a flowerpot and texted a friend to ask her to come to walk the
dog once the sun was up. Then I grabbed Don's medical records
and a sweater and followed the ambulance.

The X-rays showed that Don had fractured another disk in
his back, so they kept him overnight. I asked the doctor NOT to
give him oxycodone and stayed until Don was asleep. He was
able to come home the next day but was not supposed to get out
of bed without help. The only good thing about this latest ca-
lamity was that the hospital sent another Medicare nurse to
evaluate Don. I had told Don's primary doctor my concerns. He
merely said that if it was dementia, we could do nothing about
it. It was best to cope with the symptoms. This nurse talked to
me and Don, looked at my notes and recommended a physical
therapist and a mental evaluation. At last, a medical professional was concerned about his diminishing cognition!

The physical therapist was excellent. Over the next two years, we became friends. Every time Don went to the ER and was admitted to the hospital, she came to see him. When the six weeks of care were over, she would wave and laugh, "See you the next crisis!" The mental evaluator gave Don a short cognitive test and told me privately that a neurologist should evaluate him. At first, Don refused to go, but I pitched a good ole southern hissy fit; the boys called him and recommended that he go, and finally, Don gave in. We scheduled a complete examination and a cognitive test for dementia.

What I Learned:

1. People living with dementia are often delusional, confused, and scared. They sometimes react to their caregivers with hostility and even aggression. I found that the more I tried to "remind" Don to take his medication, be careful in the backyard, and drink his prune juice, the more annoyed and defensive he became. "You are always telling me what to do!" It doesn't help to get angry. Try to hand your LO the pills with a glass of juice and stand there until he takes them. Try saying, "It makes me less worried if you use the walker when you walk Recon.". Distraction, humor, and a friendly tone of voice all help. My mantra became Jimmy Buffett's lyric, "If we couldn't laugh, we would all go insane!"

The LBD Association has a Facebook group that anyone can join. It's helpful to see how others handle situations that you are experiencing. Recently a member posted that she had found an acronym to help her remember the best way to help manage her LO's condition. READ. Don't try to Reason, Explain, Argue, or Deny. Do try to Respond, Engage, Adapt, and Distract.

Another member quoted from a book she had recently read, "No one ever won an argument with a dementia patient."

People with Lewy Body Dementia often have delusions and "waking" dreams. When they wake up, they think their dream is reality. Once Don woke up and told me, "Get my good suit and dress shoes ready. The CIA is sending a car to pick me up for a secret mission." He smiled slyly at me and continued, "I can't tell you anymore."

I replied, "I understand. I have 'no need to know.' Let's have breakfast first." By the time he had eaten his pancakes and sausage, he had forgotten everything. I couldn't help but smile. The super CIA agent, shaken-not-stirred, international spy, was sitting in his lift chair with a plastic bib and syrup on his chin.

In her book, "The Alzheimer's Disease Caregiver's Handbook," Dr. Sally W Burbank suggests that telling your LO the absolute truth isn't helpful in some situations. For example, if your mother continually asks when her husband is coming home. It merely makes her sad or agitated to remind her that he died two years ago. She recommends that you say something like, "Dad had to work late tonight. Why don't we go bake him some cookies?" She calls this a "therapeutic lie." I found that I had to use this technique often as Don's condition got worse.

2. Put a note in big letters on the refrigerator: "Medical records are in the folder on top of the refrigerator." List all your LO's doctors and their phone numbers. Ensure you update the list of your LO's meds if they change and note any allergies and medical conditions he has. Give the names of your emergency contacts and neighbors who might help. I also kept a copy of our advanced directives in the notebook.

3. Change the alarm code on all exits, lock all guns in a cabinet and hide the key, and put knives and sharp objects on the top shelf where your LO can't see them. Move sharp tools and electric equipment to a safe place if you can. Lock the tools in a toolbox. Once Don tried to hit me with a hammer when I attempted to escort him out of the garage and back to bed. He thought I was a burglar.

4. Meet with a trusted financial advisor. Caring for a LO at home or in a facility is very expensive. Now is the time to develop a plan. It might be prudent to start your own checking account and put most of your income there. I put most of our bills on automatic payment and changed the password for the accounts.

Don would forget where he put his shampoo, toothpaste, notepaper, etc., and then buy more when we went to Walmart. I "lost" his credit cards and told him he could use mine.

5. "Sundowning" refers to increased confusion and agitation, often occurring in the early evening. Some people become frightened or aggressive; some hallucinate. No one knows precisely what causes sundowning, but experts think the sleep-wake cycle in the brain is disturbed.
They suggest keeping your LO active and awake during the day, turning on a night light in the bedroom, watching relaxing TV shows, or playing soothing music before bedtime. You can also try limiting fluids before bedtime to minimize trips to the bathroom. I put a sensor mat under Don's sheets that sent out an alarm whenever he got out of bed.

6. Ask a caregiver or a nurse to demonstrate the best way to help your LO if they have balance issues. The Medicare physical therapist suggested that I walk behind Don and use a gait belt that is placed around his waist. I would hold on to that, and it kept him from falling forward. I've seen a little 120-pound woman help a 160-pound man out of a chair. If you do it wrong, you can hurt yourself or cause both of you to fall. Ask a nurse or therapist to demonstrate the correct method. Now might be the time to get rid of that old recliner and purchase a good lift chair. As the LBD progresses, it will become indispensable.

7. Many items are available to help disabled people, from Alexa to pill boxes that buzz when it's time to take your meds. My sons always sent me ads about a new item they thought would help. However, Don quickly got to the point where he couldn't operate his phone, much less use a smartwatch! He took off and lost the ID bracelet I gave him, could not remember how to operate the little CD player I had bought, and forgot Alexa's name. An item that did help me tremendously was a mat that fits under his sheets with an alarm that went off whenever Don got out of bed. That way, I knew when he was up and wandering. Ramps and grab bars at all the doors, a jazzy red walker with USMC stickers, colorful plastic mugs, and dishes helped.

8. Don could still read, even if he couldn't follow the plot of a book. So, I made bright, cheerful signs saying BATHROOM or LAUNDRY. I put neon yellow tape at the edge of the patio and on the front steps. We labeled the individual prune juice jars by the day of the week. A bright red basket for his wallet, phone, hearing aids, and favorite flashlight was purchased. I put a neon blue plastic cup in the bathroom, and every night, we'd take out his dental plates and soak them overnight. After Don went to bed, I would search the house and find his hearing aids,

31

cellphone, wallet, etc. Then I would return them to their proper place. That saved time and stress in the morning.

9. As the disease progressed, Don became increasingly stiff and uncoordinated. He found it difficult to get in and out of bed. I would hold his hands and help him step backward until he felt the bed behind his knees. Then I would remind him to sit down. Once he sat comfortably on the bed, I helped him lean back onto the pillow. Then I would pick up his legs and place them on the bed. We reversed the procedure to get him up. Because he did get up at night, we ordered a hospital bed with a railing from the U.S. Department of Veteran Affairs (VA). The barriers helped Don pull himself up and kept him from rolling out of bed.

10. Don had always been physically fit. He ran three miles daily and went to the gym several times a week. Every morning he did his routine of push-ups and pull-ups. Now he had two compressed disk fractures, and his balance and coordination continued to decline. So, he had to stop his exercise routine. The physical therapist showed us a series of exercises we could do at the kitchen sink. Don could hold on to the counter, and I walked behind him. At first, he made fun of the "silly" exercises she suggested, but I think he realized they helped. We also joined a chair exercise group offered in our community. It was primarily women over 65, but they made Don feel right at home. Even then, he could still do ten good Marine Corps push-ups. So, our fearless exercise leader often ended the session with "OK, Don. Show us how it's done!" And Don would drop and pump out ten push-ups. As his physical strength and coordination worsened, I would sit in front of him while he was in the recliner, and we would do arm and leg exercises to music.

Many studies indicate that exercise helps both mentally and physically. Plus, it helped Don sleep at night.

11. Show your LO that you still love and respect them. We would have a glass of wine on the patio before supper and talk about places we had been or activities we enjoyed. I watched his favorite TV shows with him, and we went for long rides to get a Starbucks or ice cream. They need to know that you still care.

Brown Leaves

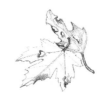

Anger, rage, denial
Pain, fear, and sorrow
I scream, "It's not fair!"

The leaves turn brown and start to crumble; pieces are whisked away by the winter wind. And Don continued to lose parts of his mind, bit by bit.

Our first trip to the neurologist went very smoothly. I filled out the new patient forms early and attached my medical and behavioral notes. So, when we met with the PA, she and the doctor already had a good idea of what was happening. The pretty little physician's assistant addressed most of her questions directly to Don. I positioned myself behind him so I could shake my head at the PA when he answered a question incorrectly. She would then ask him to clarify or ask me. Don didn't seem to be upset at all; part of the time, they were discussing UGA football!

She recommended a complete physical and brain scan to identify any problems or concerns that might be causing his symptoms. Then she set a date for a neurological doctor to give Don a cognitive test and asked us if we would like to see a psychiatrist. Don immediately and emphatically said, "NO!" I agreed because I couldn't see him discussing problems with a stranger. The PA didn't push. It was only much later that I discovered that the psychiatrist is the physician that usually determines what medications a dementia patient should take! I wish the PA had explained that.

All of the tests came back normal for Don's age. He was no longer taking oxycodone or tramadol for pain. We had changed our primary physician to a geriatric doctor, and she recommended Tylenol 3 twice a day. It seemed to help, and Don was sleeping better at night.

I was feeling hopeful. Maybe we could identify the cause of Don's hallucinations and mental decline. Perhaps it was caused by last year's trauma and the pain meds. Then we had the two-hour test for dementia. The examiner was a young, tan, slim man who looked like he belonged to the Athens cycling culture. Later I found out that, yes, he did ride his bike to work every day. Again, I had sent him every bit of information, including the recent physical examinations, so he was fully informed of Don's medical history.

He started chatting, asking us about our jobs, if we were from Athens, etc. He was charming, and I could see Don become less belligerent by the minute. When he found out Don was a retired major in the Marine Corps and had a Ph.D. from UGA, he laughingly asked if he should address him as Major or Doctor Lohmeier. Don said that the students in his classes called him Major Doc.

Then he told me he would like me to stay and watch the testing so I would be aware of what happened. Don sat at a little table facing the doctor, and I had a chair behind him. The test was brutal. It included memory and problem-solving questions; activities such as drawing the face of a clock and connecting a maze of numbers and letters. I could tell Don did well on the vocabulary and recalling basic facts. He knew who president was, the date, etc., but he couldn't do any spatial perception puzzles or problem-solving activities. He couldn't seem to follow the instructions or organize his thoughts. I was so glad I was behind him because I couldn't help crying. It broke my heart to see him struggle to do a simple puzzle. I knew Don was humiliated and upset.

After the test was over, Don just walked out to the car. I stayed to talk to the doctor, who said he would have the results in the next few days. He suggested I take Don out to dinner and try to distract him. When I got to the car, Don just looked out the window, and when I asked him where he would like to go eat, he said, "It doesn't matter." It was a sad little meal. There was no way I could distract him, and he would not talk about the test. He merely said, "I should have tried harder."
All I could say was," I love you. We'll work it out."

Fortunately, the next few days were sunny and warm, and we could take walks and go to the neighborhood picnic. We had a little Pomeranian mongrel we had adopted from the Humane Society, and he was a blessing. Don had named him "Recon" because when we got him, he loved to race around the yard, checking for intruders – cats, squirrels, deer, chipmunks…. We both loved him, but he was Don's buddy. Before Don became sick, he would take Recon with him to the gym. The owner put the dog in a little room with a doggy gate, and Recon could greet everyone. They ran together, played ball together, and

Recon went everywhere in the front seat of Don's truck with his head hanging out the window.

Our sons teased Don that he loved Recon so much because the friendly little mongrel was quite a "chick magnet"! Recon had always napped on Don's lap while Don watched TV. But now, the dog wouldn't let Don out of his sight. He followed him everywhere, and if Don sat down, Recon was in his lap. He started the tender but somewhat annoying habit of licking Don all over. Recon began sleeping at the foot of Don's bed and barking when Don went someplace without him. I felt that Recon recognized something was wrong and wanted to help. I remembered the old Snoopy comic in which Snoopy said, "My mom could lick anything well." Recon was trying.

This period of Don's illness was challenging. We knew something was wrong but didn't have a clear plan on what to do. I was so frightened and angry. Why Don? He had done everything right. He was healthy and physically fit. He was mentally active and socially involved. He kept asking, "What did I do wrong?"

One evening he said, "Teddie, we have to talk." He tried to tell me what he felt. "It's like my head is filled with little people holding signs saying, "Look at me, pay attention to me. Listen to what I'm saying." He looked at me with tears in his eyes. "I can't focus on anything!" "I can't DO anything!"

I held his hand, told him we would figure it out, and that I was always there for him and loved him unconditionally. When he took a nap, I went out into the backyard and cried and cried. "It's NOT fair!"

On the advice of a friend who had been a hospice nurse, I went to counseling. The first session was beneficial. The psychologist was friendly and comforting. I had been calm and reassuring because I didn't want to frighten Don or our sons. But I didn't know this lady, and I just vented! I expressed the anger, fear, and guilt I felt when I lost my temper with Don. I also shared my frustration that I couldn't fix it! She just reflected and nodded. I finally stopped crying and apologized to her for my meltdown. She smiled and said, "It is perfectly ok. My son says that I help people cry for a living." It felt good to laugh.

But then, she asked me why I felt guilty. I explained that sometimes I blamed Don for getting sick. I had given up so many activities that I loved. We could no longer go dancing or travel. We didn't go places with our friends because Don felt anxious and humiliated about his inability to retrieve the correct word and frequent need to urinate. I felt that my days were reduced to just being a caretaker. I had been robbed of my life. The therapist suggested that I go home and write down everything I missed and bring it back to our next session. I went home and wrote a long list: line dancing, singing with the community singers, painting, the Arts Council, canceling the cruise to Alaska, and sleeping at night. Then I looked at the list and laughed. I had left out that my parents had never gotten me a pony! Suddenly compared to what Don was going through, my sacrifices seemed trivial. I canceled the therapist.

My son, David, had been helping me with research and suggestions. We were actively pursuing the idea that Don's condition might have been caused by exposure to Agent Orange during his two years in Vietnam. Greg, Dave, Mel (Dave's wife), and I called, wrote letters, had interviews, and sent emails – the VA bureaucracy was enough to make all of us crazy! Dave, who had served as an Army helicopter pilot, finally found another Army vet with a home care business. He was a tremendous help in offering practical advice.

Finally, after over a year of trying, Don was granted a small VA benefit allotment. Not for dementia but for his prostate cancer fifteen years prior. However, we received sixteen hours of caregiving help a week! I was so excited – I could go to the grocery store alone. I could get my hair cut or even play cards with friends. Don was furious. "I don't need anyone to babysit me!" he fumed. And he ran off almost every caregiver who came.

Some of the caregivers were definitely not what I expected. The caregivers I saw on TV were young, fit, cheerful, and well-trained. One young girl came to care for Don and said she was only doing this job to save up for art school. She just sat on the sofa and stared at Don. Don finally growled, "What the hell are you staring at!". She started crying and left. Another older woman came to spend the night so I could sleep. I had prepared a recliner and a table in Don's bedroom with a blanket, water, and snacks. I put a small lamp next to the chair so she could read. The caregiver came in, and I showed her the place I had prepared. She said she would rather stay in the living room and pulled out a pillow and comforter from her bag. Then she curled up on the sofa. At about two in the morning, Don walked into the guest room and woke me. He had pulled off his incontinence briefs and told me a stranger was asleep on the sofa, snoring! It took a while before we found someone we both liked!

Everyone dreads the day when they must stop driving. When it happens, you lose the freedom to pick up and go when-ever you wish. You become dependent on friends, family, Uber drivers, or public transport. Where we lived, if you didn't have a vehicle, you had to ask someone to drive you.

The psychiatric examiner finally called and asked us to come in to go over the results of Don's testing. He explained that Don still had a good vocabulary, was aware of his surround-ings, and recalled family names. However, he struggled with math, spatial perception, and problem-solving. The doctor de-clared that Don had "unspecified dementia."

I sarcastically thought, "Well, that really helps!"

Then he looked at Don and said, "I strongly recommend that you not drive anymore."

Don looked as if someone had slapped him. "I'm an excellent driver!" he stated emphatically and left.

The doctor told me that with Don's spatial perception disability, he could easily have a bad accident and hurt himself or others.

One night after dinner, I told Don the story of my dad's reluctance to give up driving. My sister told him she knew he didn't want to be responsible for killing an innocent person. Dad reluctantly agreed to surrender his license.

Don said he had only had three accidents in sixty years of driving, and only one was his fault. "I can see just fine, and I don't think my judgment is impaired!" I changed the subject, but my sons and I brought it up repeatedly over the next few weeks. Finally, I called the doctor and asked how I could get the state to revoke Don's driver's license. He directed me to the Georgia driver's license website and said that an eye doctor could recommend that Don get tested. I challenged Don to take the test. I said that if he passed, I wouldn't bother him anymore. He reluctantly agreed.

We showed up at the driver's license bureau, and they directed us to a small room. Again, I was told that it would be good for me to watch so I would understand the results. The examiner tested Don's eyesight, peripheral vision, reflexes, and spatial perception. He did not do well. When the examiner reviewed the results with him, he tried arguing with her. "I can see fine. I don't even need glasses!" She explained that the main problem was not visual acuity but spatial perception and reflex time. Don left very upset.

A week later, we received a letter from the driver's license department asking that Don surrender his license. They said he had failed the test and was no longer qualified to drive. Don was devastated. He went into his study and closed the door. I was terribly concerned about what he might do. So, after a moment, I opened the door and sat beside him. Don looked up and whispered, "I'm falling apart. Little by little, my life is being taken from me."

I tried to make him laugh by reminding him of all the years we only had one car, and I had to ride my bike to the grocery store. But there was nothing I could say to help. So, I went and cooked supper.

Things did not get better. One morning I took Don to our community pool, thinking water therapy would help us. Don had been a scuba instructor, and we were both qualified divers. But Don acted as if he were afraid of the water. He wouldn't go underwater and seemed unsteady, just trying to walk back and forth across the pool. He finally said that he had to go the bathroom, so we got out, and he went into the men's room. When he came out, he was wrapped in his towel. Then I realized he was holding his bathing suit! I ran over and hissed, "Why did you take off your suit?" "It was wet.", he stated. People were drifting in for water aerobics, so I wrapped the towel tightly around his bare bottom and hustled him out to the car. We didn't go back.

Don lost everything: his wallet, his glasses, his phone. He dropped one of his hearing aids down the toilet and flushed it. I found his lower dental plate in a trash can. One day, we were in a hurry to get to a doctor's office. Getting Don dressed had taken me forever, and it was pouring rain outside. I got Don settled in the car and jumped in. My keys weren't in my purse. I couldn't believe it. I always left them in my purse. I climbed out into the rain, ran to the front door, and reached under the flowerpot for the spare keys. They weren't there! I knew I had a spare set in my locked file box. I just had to get into the house.

41

So, I went to the back of the house and checked the window to Don's bathroom. I always left it cracked for more ventilation. I managed to get it up, pried off the screen, climbed through the window, raced to the front door to turn off the alarm system, and went and got my spare key. I was soaking wet, I had a tear in my shirt, but I scrambled back to the car and started it up. Don asked me where I had been. "I told you.", I said. "I couldn't find my car keys."

"Do you mean these keys? "He said, pulling my old keys out of his pocket. I was still shaking when we got to the doctor!

We were invited to a 50's Sock Hop sponsored by the Silver Sneakers group at the community center. Several good friends were going, so I thought we could handle it. Don wore a vintage flight jacket, a white T-shirt with a cigarette pack stuck in the rolled-up sleeve, and I wore jeans and bobby socks, Don's white dress shirt with the sleeves rolled up, a scarf around my neck, and a high school ring around my neck. It was fun. We loved the music, laughing with friends, and enjoying the burgers and milkshakes. We danced a few slow numbers, but Don couldn't manage the shag (this was the man who did a tap dance routine at our local charity Dancing with the Stars event). As we left, he looked back and remarked that he needed to go back and retake dance lessons. He stopped and grabbed my hand. "It's not too late, is it? I can still do it?"

While we had become familiar with the hallucinations, Don now started having more intense "waking" dreams. He would dream he was called in for duty and would get up at two in the morning and try to get out of the house to join his regiment. I couldn't explain that it wasn't happening. To him, it was real. I'd say, "Well, I guess the escort is a little late. Why don't we have some hot chocolate and wait for him". Generally, I could distract him and get him back in bed.

One night he was very constipated and found the mineral oil I had hidden and drank half a bottle. By midnight, he had cramps and diarrhea. He would wake up every hour, and I would help him to the bathroom. I was so exhausted that one time I didn't hear him get up. I woke when I heard the door alarm go off. I ran to the foyer and found Don naked and dribbling feces. He was trying to get outside. I answered the emergency call and told the operator we were not being robbed while I tried to get Don to hold a towel under his bare bottom. He just threw it down and kept lurching around the house, dropping clumps of stinky poop. I couldn't make him stop or go to the bathroom. He kept saying that he had to find the blue bucket. No matter what I did, he would shove me aside and keep searching.

I finally just flopped down on the sofa and watched. When Don eventually fell into the recliner exhausted, I was able to coax him into the bathroom. I cleaned him up, helped him put on a pair of incontinence briefs, and gave him a Tylenol #3. Then while he slept, I cleaned feces off the floor, the rug, and the recliner. I pulled a rocking chair up to the door of his room so he couldn't leave his room without waking me and collapsed. The next day I called a professional cleaner to sanitize the entire house. Eventually, Don told me his family didn't have indoor plumbing when he was a child on the farm. In the freezing winters of Nebraska, he used a little blue bucket instead of walking to the outhouse. He had dreamed he was a little ten-year-old boy.

Even with the cognitive decline, the hallucinations, and the waking dreams, I felt I could care for him at home. I had someone come twice a week to spend the night so I could get eight hours of blessed sleep. We found some caregivers who could entertain Don by playing music or looking at scrapbooks so that I could get out of the house. My neighbors were wonderful.

Some of the gentlemen in the neighborhood would come by in the afternoon, have a beer and tell war stories. One creative lady told Don that she would be babysitting her grandson that weekend and needed to learn how to make paper airplanes to keep him busy. She and Don spent a fun afternoon making and flying paper airplanes while I napped! A dear man across the street told me I could call him night or day if I needed help moving Don or picking him up. And I did!

It was difficult to have a conversation with Don. He would often use the incorrect word. For example, he told a friend that she looked "livid" rather than "lovely." He would become confused and describe how he fell off a bird's wing when describing our experience with gliders in Colorado. He would mix up items he heard on the news: "The Pope was arrested for computer hacking. "I could generally decode the message and translate. But sometimes, we would have to smile when Don smiled and look sympathetic when Don seemed upset. However, with the support of family, our medical team, and friends, I felt we could manage and planned to stay in our new community for a long while.

Then came COVID-19.

We were living in an "over fifty" community. The residents had grown up with the threat of the Cold War, Vietnam, 9/11, and global warming. The idea of a new type of flu didn't bother us much. We wore our masks, kept a safe distance apart when we walked our dogs, closed the exercise class, and canceled the New Year's Eve party. But we also did chalk paintings on the sidewalk, left chicken soup on neighbor's front porches, and posted funny pictures on Facebook. I even made watercolor Pandemic poetry cards and left them in my friends' mailboxes.

We didn't think the crisis would last long. But reality soon set in.

My caregivers started to call and cancel their visits. One had no childcare; another had a sick mother and yet another had an immune defective son. I only had one helper, a dear lady who worked part-time as a pharmacy assistant and already had her Covid vaccination. She came at night twice a week – but I was lucky if I could get anyone to help during the day. The isolation took its toll. We would walk Recon and wave at friends. I started setting a rocking chair out in the afternoon so Don could have a beer and yell at folks across the street.

Our sons would visit and deliver groceries or talk to us from the curb. The youngest, Dave, was in Arkansas and he and his wife would facetime us on the phone. All of them would text, send pictures or funny cartoons to let us know we were not alone.

However, Don and I both became cranky and quick to snap at each other. His urologist had suggested that we stop doing urinary surgical dilations because there was no room at the hospitals. Instead, Don was supposed to use a self-catheter once a day.

He often forgot the sanitary precautions the nurse had tried to drill into us and would not let me help him. He had several urinary infections, and I was afraid that he would become resistant to antibiotics. So, I insisted that I help when he used the catheter. First, I posted a colorful sign over the toilet listing the steps to take, starting with WASH YOUR HANDS!

One day, I lost it and snatched the catheter from Don's hands. I began barking orders. "Wash your hands with hot water and put on the plastic gloves! Don't touch the toilet seat with your gloved hands!" "Now, you must change gloves!" "Foot, just let me do it." So, you had two very annoyed adults in the bathroom wrestling over the catheter.

"I can do this," yelled Don. "I know what to do!" Then looking at the sign with instructions, he asked me, "So, where's my penis?"

The emergency rooms of hospitals in town became dangerous places to go. People were coughing and sneezing, and there were beds in the hallways. So, when Don developed another impacted bowel, I had to do what the ER doctor and nurse did. I un-impacted it. Again, I had to laugh at the picture of a grown man lying sideways on the bed, yelling every time I got near him. "It hurts. Call the EMTs!" But I was able to remove the hard feces, clean him up afterward and get him settled on the patio with the dog and a beer. Then I had a nice, quiet meltdown!

One afternoon, Don was so depressed. He was tired of TV, didn't want to listen to music, refused to look at a scrapbook – I couldn't think of anything to do. He told me that he missed our old life so much. It was four in the afternoon, but I called and found our favorite Italian place open. People could still come to sit on the patio if they wore masks. We took Recon and ordered wine, bacon spinach crostini, and water and cheese sticks for the dog. We drank wine, told stories about the good old days, had Recon do tricks for the cute little server, and relaxed. We stayed until the patio started filling up. As we drove home, we listened to jazz on the radio and watched the sunset. I still cherish that memory.

It was December, and it was cold and grey outside. Don and I were arguing about the caregivers. (Note: never argue with someone with dementia – you can't win!) I was at my wit's end because every time I managed to get someone to come in, Don was so rude and uncooperative that they refused to return! One dear man kept trying. He had been a caregiver all his life and was kind and helpful. I know all the older ladies that he worked with adored him. He bothered Don to death. Don said he "hovered" and got in the way when he tried to move. He told me repeatedly that he wanted to get rid of him. I finally gave in and told Charley that Don was a cantankerous old man and didn't like anyone. I gave Charley $100, thanked him profusely, and told him we couldn't use him anymore.

When I told Don what I had done, he looked at me and said, "Well, that's cold. Firing a guy just before Christmas!"

I just sat on the sofa and rocked back and forth, laughing, and crying.

Don looked perplexed and said, "Honey, you look upset. How can I help?"

Besides washing dirty sheets daily, cleaning the bathroom every time Don used it, walking the dog, cleaning the house, cooking, helping Don dress, using the catheter, and walking to the recliner, I also had to entertain him. If I sat down to read the paper, he just stood before me, staring. When I looked up, he would say, "My phone doesn't work." or "I can't find my wallet."

I helped him make scrapbooks, listened to old records, and watched reruns of Bonanza. He couldn't read, hated card games, and disliked playing catch. He wanted to do projects. He'd sit next to me and say we needed to plan the Marine Corps birthday ball or the Lion's Club annual car show. He'd want me to drive him out to the airport so he could talk to the manager about the airshow. He was bored, and I was going crazy.

One day I found him taking apart the voltmeter because it "wouldn't work right." He wanted to check all of the batteries in the house. I finally got a box of batteries and a flashlight. I showed him that he could put the batteries in the flashlight and turn it on to see if they worked. That lasted about ten minutes. He kept putting the batteries in upside down. When I just ran out of things for him to do, I'd put him in the car, and we'd drive to the Dairy Queen and get ice cream or go to the airport and watch the airplanes take off and land. I couldn't do anything by myself.

I was fortunate in that I could talk to some friends, my sons, and my sister about the changes in Don and how I could cope. My sister and I texted almost every day. I shared heartbreaking and funny things with her. But one thing I could never share with anyone was my changing sexual feelings. Despite my best efforts, I could not feel the desire for a person who smelled of urine. I no longer could think of him as a lover; he was more my patient.

When Don became impotent, I felt relief. I also felt guilty and ashamed of my feelings, but it was easier to cuddle and caress. I knew he still needed to feel loved and cherished, and I did my best. And I did love him.

Don hurt his back again and struggled to get in and out of bed. I tore my gluteus medius muscle trying to get him up off the floor, and I could barely walk. With COVID still raging, Greg, our eldest son, worked from home. So, he moved into the guest room and stayed with us for a week. We took turns sleeping. We had difficulty getting Don to sleep one night, and Greg had a meeting in Atlanta the next day. So, we called Michelle, a trusted caregiver, and she came over to care for Don while we slept. At three in the morning, I heard Don yelling and Michelle trying to calm him.

Greg and I ran into the bedroom and found Don yelling and struggling while Michelle tried to keep him from falling out of bed. Don was bellowing, "Incoming fire! Take cover! Fall back!" Call for air support! Where's the goddamn Gunny?" Greg was attempting to keep Don on the bed, and I was trying to talk to him. Don tried to slug Greg and pushed me away. "My back! I've been shot. Get the medic. Is the ambassador safe?"

Finally, I leaned over and shouted, "Major Lohmeier, sir! We've called for air support, and the troops are being evacuated.

The ambassador is safe and on his way to Germany." "You've been wounded, and we must prepare you for evacuation. Please, sir, lay still so the medic can help." Miranda ran and got a Tylenol #3, and Greg lifted Don back on the bed. Everyone acted like we were in a Vietnam War movie and managed to calm Don down and get him asleep. As soon as the meds took effect, Don collapsed. We just stood there looking at him. I thought, "There's no way I can do this alone.

Not all the dreams were so dramatic. Another night, Greg and I put Don to bed after watching some old TV shows. We had just poured ourselves some wine and taken a deep breath when Don came out of the bedroom. He was in his incontinence briefs and a white T-shirt with the umbrella and hat he wore when he did his "Dancing with the Stars" routine. He cocked his hat, smiled, and said, "I'm ready." Greg and I looked at each other. "Ah, ready for what?"

"My entrance. Tell them to start my music."

We finally realized that he thought he was on the Carol Burnett show! I explained that because of COVID, they had to cancel the show until next week. Greg suggested some cookies and hot chocolate, and we all sat down. Curious, I asked, "Babe, what were you going to sing?

Don looked a bit nonplussed and then grinned. "I do better when I improvise!" We "practiced" singing old songs until he got sleepy and returned to bed.

I knew that Don needed to get a COVID-19 vaccination. However, it was almost impossible to find someplace that had a supply. Finally, I made an appointment at the VA hospital, two hours from our house. I packed the car as if we were on an expedition to Antarctica. Meds, check. Extra clothes, check.

Spare incontinence briefs, check. Urinal, in case we couldn't find a bathroom, check. Snacks check. Don liked to ride and listen to the radio, so the first hour was calm.

Then we both had to go to the bathroom, so we stopped at a small, rural gas station. I went into the men's bathroom with Don, helped him, and relieved myself. Coming out, Don said that he wanted a Diet Coke and some peanuts. His balance had worsened, so I told him to stand by the checkout counter, and I would be right back. I raced to the drink cooler and snatched up a packet of peanuts. By the time I got back to the counter, Don was gone. Frantic, I ran outside just in time to see Don fall backward off the curb – into the arms of a young black man! The stranger gently helped Don back onto the sidewalk and walked with him over to me. I was relieved and said, "Thank you so much!" Deon introduced himself and offered to get Don settled in the car while I paid for my purchases. When I returned, Deon said he and Don had been discussing the Marine Corps. Deon had seen the sticker on our car and told Don, "I just returned from Afghanistan." Then he asked me, "Could I know your first names? I will add you to our prayer list." There are good people in this world.

One afternoon while Don was napping, I sat down and made a list of our problems. Don was using a self-catheter every day and suffered from frequent urinary infections. His back was still very painful from his fractured compressed disks. Don's balance and coordination were poor, and his cognitive abilities had deteriorated, so he could no longer write or understand what he read. His short-term memory was deficient, and he suffered from hallucinations and delusions! We couldn't get reliable help, I couldn't lift him anymore because of my shredded gluteus medius, and because of COVID, neighbors, and friends couldn't come by. I could only talk to doctors through Zoom meetings and couldn't even leave Don to go to the grocery store.

Either my middle son, Brad, delivered them, or I would load the dog and Don into the car and pick them up at the store. I decided that I had to look for a memory care facility. I felt so guilty – how could I put my husband in a facility?

Again, I turned to my sons for help. Our youngest, Dave, was out of state, but he helped tremendously with financial advice, research, and cheering me up with phone calls and Calvin and Hobbes cartoons. Brad told me I could move in with him. Greg helped me with Don's physical care and contributed his considerable legal knowledge. We searched the web for health and safety records for memory care facilities, compared staff-to-patient ratios, and called to find availability and cost. It was time-consuming and frustrating. And whenever I even mentioned it, Don said he would not go!

We tried to explain that I couldn't care for him because of my bad back and a shredded hip muscle. But he just said he would not move into a facility. It was the hardest thing I ever did, but I contacted his primary physician, and she filled out the paperwork saying that Don needed to be placed in a memory care setting. We found a facility near Brad's house and had the admitting nurse come by and interview Don. She gave him the same little test that the other medical staff had used, but Don didn't remember the questions. He couldn't draw the clock, remember the names of his grandchildren, and became confused when the nurse asked him questions about his past. He definitely qualified for memory/dementia care placement. I put the house up for sale and started the very familiar process of packing up, giving away, and disposing of stuff! Both Don and I were depressed, upset, and very stressed!

Fortunately, the week before Don was scheduled to move into memory care, I received some good news. Months ago, I sent a packet to the Georgia Military Veterans Hall of Fame nominating Don for consideration. I had copied awards, commendations, and citations. I wrote to USMC headquarters and requested an official list of Don's service and medals. I asked leaders of the community and civic groups to which Don belonged to write letters detailing his service. I edited Don's bio and asked the local Military Officers Association to sponsor him. In March 2021, I received the news that Don had been accepted for consideration!

Because of COVID, I couldn't plan a reception and party for Don. So, I asked a friend to make me a shadow box with Don's medals and Bronze Star for valor. Two members of the Military Association offered to present the certificate and the shadow box to Don. We decided to hold the little ceremony on the front porch of our community clubhouse. Instead of a party, I asked friends, neighbors, colleagues, club members, and family to drive by one afternoon, honk their horns, and wave to Don.

Don was presented the certificate, and then a long parade of cars decorated with balloons and banners drove past with people waving, honking, and shouting, "Congratulations!" Don wasn't sure what was happening, but he knew they were honoring him. It was the best sendoff we could have had. We planned to move him into a memory care facility the following week.

What I Learned.

1. I always prided myself on being strong and resilient. Once Don and I figured out that during his career in the Marines, he was deployed away from home over half the time. I cared for the kids, paid the bills, mowed the lawn, etc. But becoming a caregiver is different. Before I always hoped that things would get better; Don would come home from Vietnam, the puppy would be housebroken, and the youngest boy would start school. But with dementia, you knew things would only get

worse. I had to live the Serenity Prayer" Lord, give me the strength to change what can be changed, accept what cannot be changed, and the wisdom to know the difference." I had to learn to seek help, find humor where possible, and try to care for myself. As every book I read said, "You must put your own oxygen mask on first."

2. Telling your LO that he can no longer drive is one of the most emotional things a caregiver will encounter. No one wants to lose his independence, and most dementia patients don't realize they are a risk to themselves and others. If your LO won't give up the keys willingly, you can enlist the help of an authority figure such as a doctor, police officer, or minister to talk to your LO. If your LO can still understand, explain that if he is driving with a diagnosis of dementia and causes an accident, he will be liable and may have to pay damages. See if you can get the driver's license formally revoked. Then keep the keys locked up!

3. As your LO's health and cognition decline, you will probably need help to care for him. Reach out to family, friends, church groups, and civic organizations to see if they can assist you. Contact your local Council on Aging in your community and see if there is a senior citizen's center where you can leave your LO for a few hours. Meals on Wheel can deliver one meal a day. Check into Home Health agencies, but check with the Better Business Bureau, your doctors, and friends who might have used them to ensure they are reputable and have trained and reliable caregivers. Assisted living communities provide housing, meals, medication supervision, and help with daily living. Most also have services such as daily activities and transportation to doctor's appointments. The downside is that rooms are usually small, and if you need more medical care, you have to move to

a memory care unit or a nursing home. Ask if they allow you to bring Kitty or Fido!

4. Our first choice was to move to a smaller house in an "over fifty" community. The VA had awarded Don 16 hours a week of home health care, and we loved the community. If you choose to move into a senior community, read the homeowner's association guide carefully before signing the contract. We had to sell our truck because the HOA required that all vehicles be kept in the garage overnight, and our truck wouldn't fit! But after living there for three years, we had to find a memory care facility.

5. At this point, our doctors hadn't definitively labeled Don's condition as LBD. The only way to confidently diagnose the condition is to examine the brain after death! However, given Don's symptoms: fluctuating degrees of cognitive and memory decline, hallucinations, sundowning, delusions, intense "waking" dreams, loss of his sense of smell, and poor balance and coordination, they agreed with me that it didn't seem like Alzheimer's. This is important because some common medications given to dementia patients to help their cognition or emotional state can be harmful to LBD patients. Drugs such as Haldol can make symptoms worse.

LBD is often confused with Parkinson's disease. Many experts believe that Lewy Body Dementia and Parkinson's are just two different presentations of the same condition. If the tremors, loss of balance, and physical problems occur first and dementia at a later stage, it's diagnosed as Parkinson's. If cognitive and emotional issues are present before tremors and physical changes, it's LBD. Talk to your doctors to make sure they have experience with LBD patients.

6. Every patient is different, so caregivers must deal creatively with their LOs' conditions. Tips for caregivers can be found in many books and online. The LBD Association has a Facebook group you can join and ask others how they handled situations. As Don was falling a lot, I had an occupational nurse come to the house and recommend things I could do to make things safer. I gave away the beautiful carpet we bought in Turkey because Don kept catching his toe on the edge and falling forward. I took the locks of every door in the house (except those leading outside) so Don couldn't lock himself inside the bathroom or study. I purchased an upholstered bed table, so he wouldn't hurt himself getting out of bed. I got him a medical ID to wear and put an emergency call card in his wallet. I asked the neighbors to call me if they saw him walking alone in the neighborhood. In the later stages of the disease, I gave my eldest son our sleep number bed and turned the master bedroom into a hospital room. I slept in a twin bed, and Don slept in a hospital bed near the bathroom. We organized the room so supplies such as incontinence briefs, gloves, sanitary wipes, and disinfectants were readily available.

I closed the closet door each night and hung bells on the bedroom door. The goals were to make it as safe as possible and easy for Don to find the toilet!

7. Entertaining or finding activities your LO can still enjoy is daunting. Don's hobbies were all outdoor activities, and he could no longer fly his plane, run, go to the gym, or help at community events. Don had forgotten the rules to card games and didn't enjoy doing puzzles. He loved music, so we played records and enjoyed the Music Channel on TV. I tried to find old musicals to watch and even arranged some sing-a-longs

with neighbors. Sometimes I asked him to help me fold clothes, set the table, or sort the junk drawer. (Just be prepared to redo the work if necessary). I asked him to join me in doing chair exercises to music. We'd take the dog for walks and drive out to pick up the pizza to get out of the house. Again, ask others for ideas.

8. Once you decide you can no longer care for your LO at home, you should assess how much money you will need to place him in memory care. In 2021 the average cost of memory care for Georgia was over $6000 a month and didn't include medications, personal care items, incontinence briefs, haircuts, dentists, eye doctors, etc. It took Don's pension and the benefit he received from the VA to cover just the monthly fee. My retirement wouldn't cover all the other expenses, so I sold our house and moved in with my son.

9. Finding a good memory care facility is a daunting task. You can use search engines on your computer to find places near you. However, the websites show pictures of smiling and laughing seniors, beautiful entrance areas with fireplaces, grand pianos, and tall windows open to manicured grounds. The text describes spacious rooms, activity-filled days, and gourmet dining. You call the information number and feel like you're talking to a salesman, not a caregiver. But there are ways to get essential facts. If you have a senior citizen council in your area, call them for recommendations. Ask friends and family for reviews. I had a friend who was a volunteer ombudsman for assisted living and nursing homes, and she gave me advice. Your doctor, nurses, and caregivers who come to your home can provide unbiased opinions. Also, each state has a website that lists facts on each registered facility listing ratings on cleanliness, safety problems, staff-to-patient ratios, etc. I made a chart

comparing facilities near my son's house so we could make an informed decision. Then, of course, you must wait until there is an opening. We were fortunate. After a few months of research, we found a highly rated, new assisted living/memory care community only twelve miles from my son's home. The hardest part was getting Don to go there.

Withered Leaves

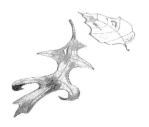

Is a slow leaching of life
Every day, joy fades

Sometimes a golden Indian Summer brightens late autumn. The few last colorful leaves on the trees sparkle before they, too, turn brown and wither. I knew Don was entering the final stages of LBD. All I could do was keep him comfortable and cherish the few incidents of laughter and happiness.

My sons all came to help move Don into the memory care unit. Dave had flown down from Arkansas, and Brad had taken off from work. Greg helped me complete the volumes of paperwork. I had gotten Don all the appropriate vaccines and signed the myriad forms. Don didn't even ask why we were moving his bed, chest of drawers, and recliner into the U-Haul truck. He didn't seem to notice that we had taken some of his favorite pictures, awards, and memorabilia off the walls of his study. He was too busy greeting the neighbors who stopped by. Bless them; no one said "Goodbye." They just reminded him of some good times we had together or said they hoped to see him again soon. The young lady who had been cutting our hair for the last two years even came over to our house with her clippers and bib to trim his hair and beard. Don still retained the "social graces." Even when he couldn't remember the name of the person he was talking to, he'd say, "Thank you for stopping by." Or "I so enjoyed your visit."

The next day after going out for lunch, the boys and I drove him to his new home. The facility was relatively new and attractive, with the ubiquitous large fireplace and piano in the entry. The grounds were well-kept, and the receptionist and director were smiling and cheerful. Assisted living residents were reading or watching TV. Some were strolling the sidewalks in the fenced courtyard. Then we were ushered into the memory care unit.

The TV was on, and three aides were there to greet us. The unit had room for 25 patients, and because of COVID, there were several empty rooms. The walls were painted in a light color with cheerful pictures and shelves held games and magazines. We had arranged Don's private room, so the bed was under the window and the recliner faced the open door. His familiar pictures and awards hung on the walls, and the large TV was on the chest of drawers. However, the residents were wandering aimlessly or sitting at tables staring at their hands. One little lady stood by the locked door to the courtyard pounding on it. "I want to go home," she said over and over. There was a malaise of sorrow and hopelessness everywhere.

We introduced Don to the director and aides. He just smiled and nodded. We showed him (and the aides) how to operate the

TV and where his clothes, etc., were located. Finally, looking very apprehensive, the boys hugged Don and said they had to go. Don smiled brightly and replied, "Just a minute, I'll get my coat."

My sons looked at me in a panic, and I motioned that they should leave. I asked Don if he wanted to walk around the grounds, and he agreed. I stayed until dinner and told him I had to go home and walk Recon. He immediately got up and said, "Let's go." I gently told him that he had to stay, that the nurse and the aides would take care of him, and that I would return later. He just looked stunned, and I quickly left. I cried all the way home.

The memory care director had briefed me earlier and said that I shouldn't come back to visit him for two weeks so Don could adjust to living there. I remarked that I didn't think that would work, but we could try. She just patted my hand and said, "He'll be fine. We do this all the time." I received a phone call at about midnight. The nurse from memory care told me that Don was distraught and demanded to talk to me. She handed the phone to Don, and he exploded. "Teddie, you have to get me out of here! They are violating my civil rights – holding me prisoner! You need to call Greg and get me a lawyer right now. I can't stay locked up with these retarded people! I mean it. If you can't get me out, I'm going to break the window and climb the god damned wall!"

I just listened, and when he took a breath, I spoke as calmly as possible.

"Babe, I understand that you're really upset. But it's late, and I can't get hold of anyone right now. Are you OK? Have you had your meds?"

"I'm not taking anything from these people. They are going to drug me!"

"Don, I will be there first thing in the morning, and we will try to work this out. But I need you to take your medicine so you can get a good night's sleep. You know I love you, and I'll be there as soon as possible."

Don took a deep breath, and I could tell he was trying not to cry. "I love you too. I'll see you in the morning."

He handed the phone to the nurse, and I told her what I had said. I told her I would be there in the morning right after breakfast. She agreed and hung up. I took two sleeping pills and tried to sleep. I have never felt so guilty or lost.

The next day I arrived at about nine with my mask, a doughnut, and a cup of cappuccino. After wandering around the facility all night, trying to find a way to escape, Don had slept through breakfast and was starving. The staff was able to order some cold cereal and fruit from the kitchen. It was a lovely day, so we took his food out to the porch and ate there. He was calmer but just as adamant that he needed to leave immediately. I explained again that I couldn't care for him at home because of my injury, and we couldn't get reliable caregivers. I also told him that I had sold the house and was planning on moving into a room at the facility as soon as I packed all our stuff. This wasn't a lie. Brad's roommate was getting married and moving out, but their new house wasn't ready yet. So, I planned to put the possessions I had left into storage and take a "respite" room in the assisted living area. However, now I was still living thirty minutes away! Don seemed to accept that he would be there alone for a while, and I left after lunch.

I immediately went to speak to the facility's director and explained that I would be coming by each day. She said that wasn't possible because the COVID numbers had gone back up, and they were not allowing visitors. I asked her what credentials you needed to be an aide. She told me they had to have experience working with dementia patients and were required to get a negative COVID test each week. I told her that I had been the lead teacher of the special education department at my school and had thirty years of experience working with learning-disabled and gifted children, with a doctorate in educational leadership. Reminding her that I had been caring for Don at home for five years, I also said I would be more than willing to get a COVID test each week. She reluctantly agreed to designate me as an "essential caregiver" for Don. I left to find a place to get a COVID test.

Unfortunately, Don did not settle into his new home peacefully. At eight o'clock the following day, the memory care director called me and told me that Don was having a psychotic episode and was throwing things and cursing the aides. I needed to come to get him at once and admit him to the psych ward at the hospital. I made it over there in fifteen minutes and rushed into the ward. Don's door was closed, and the aides said they wouldn't go in there because they feared getting injured. I cracked the door and yelled, "Don, it's me, Teddie." Then I walked in and found him sitting on the edge of his bed surrounded with plastic cups, paper pads, and pens – evidently missiles ready to be hurled at the enemy. He hugged me and said, "How did you get past the guards? We've got to get out of here!"

I sat down and held his hand. "What's going on?"

Don told me he was in a Japanese prisoner-of-war camp, and they were trying to make him talk about his regiment. "I only gave them my name, rank, and serial number.", he informed me.

I took a deep breath and explained that I had arranged for his release, and we were going to the field hospital to get him checked out, but he had to get dressed first. We walked out, Don ready to defend me if necessary. I told the director that I'd call from the hospital. She told me they had already called and checked him in. I got Don in the car, and we went through the drive-through at Wendy's to get some coffee and biscuits. I turned on his favorite radio station, and we started to the hospital. Soon Don had biscuit crumbs all over the car, was singing along with the music, and commenting about the beautiful weather.

When we got to the hospital, I tried to explain what happened. The nurse looked at the calm, happy, and sleepy man on the bed and called the memory care unit. The director said they couldn't take him back because he was a danger to her staff, and the nurse agreed to keep him overnight. I was confused and upset. Was the memory care facility refusing to care for him? What should I do? Where should I take him? The nurse said the doctor would be in to talk to me later. Don was sound asleep by this time, so I texted my sons and told them what had happened. And then I curled up in the chair next to his bed and watched him sleep.

The doctor came, listened to my story, checked Don out, and examined the medical record that I had brought with me. They decided to give him a psychological examination and observe him overnight. Don was quite happy. The food was good, the TV worked, the nurses were cheerful, and I was there tending to his every need. Because of COVID, I couldn't spend the night, so I went home to walk the dog and pack more boxes. The next day, the doctor released Don and said he did not need a psych ward placement and I should take him back to memory care. The director was not happy but welcomed us both back.

Don had two more episodes that week. They happened in the morning, right after he woke up and was still caught up in his nightmares. The second time they called me, I found him nude, sitting on the bed, looking frightened and worried. As I walked in, he cried, "Hurry, get in the magic circle. They have no power here!"

I sat down beside him, and he hugged me. When I asked him what was bothering him, he explained that the aides were members of a witches' coven. They were trying to kill him. He said that if he left the bed, bats would come and bite him, and the witches would come in muttering spells. I just listened and then said, "Well, for some reason, the spells didn't hurt me. Maybe if we make the sign of the cross and get into the bathroom, we can escape."

Don nervously agreed to try and holding our hands up in the sign of the cross, we carefully walked into the bathroom and closed the door. I cleaned him up, dressed him, and cheerfully told him I would bring Recon in the next day. Soon he was calm and ready for breakfast.

I tried to explain to the director and aids that when he had one of these "awake" dreams, it was reality for him. Saying, "It's OK, Mr. Don, let's just come out and get some nice orange juice," made him more upset. In his mind, he knew that moving out of the magic circle would be disastrous! I don't think anyone in the facility had ever experienced a patient with LBD. Alzheimer patients don't usually have hallucinations and wild acting-out dreams!

The third time Don thought that there had been a nuclear bomb attack and he had to leave the facility and find me and our family. He fought the aides when they tried to restrain him and then bit the director. This time the director called the EMTs to take Don to the hospital and then called me. When I got to the hospital, the nurses had Don restrained on the bed. It took a while to calm everyone down!

The admitting nurse explained that the memory care director had called them and said that Don was a danger to himself and others and should be placed in a psychiatric hospital. When Don got to the hospital, he was angry and upset. He kept trying to get off the bed and leave the hospital. When I could sit down and talk to Don, he was sobbing. "I thought you were dead! They wouldn't let me go find you!"

I turned on the TV news and showed him that no one was discussing an atomic attack. I suggested that perhaps it was just a nightmare. He finally went to sleep, and I could talk to the nurse. She insisted that if the memory care unit wouldn't take Don back and he had already suffered three of these psychotic events, he would be placed in a psychiatric ward. I knew that he would only get worse there!

I called Greg, a lawyer, and told him what was happening. I was close to hysterics and explained that I didn't know what to do. Could they force me to admit Don to a psychiatric ward? Within the hour, my son was there and talking to the hospital's legal department. Our other sons and daughters-in-law also made phone calls to find out our rights. The hospital agreed to allow Don to stay in his room if a family member was present, so either Greg or I was in the room for the next two days. We talked to psychiatrists, our primary doctor, other lawyers, and hospital administrators. My sister came and watched the dog and supervised the movers as they carried boxes and furniture from my storage unit into Brad's garage. Brad came home from work at 1:00 in the morning and moved furniture. Dave contacted the VA to see if they could help.

We discovered that if Don were placed in a psychiatric hospital because he was a danger to others, we couldn't check him out until the staff decided he was stabilized. Meanwhile, Don was being the model patient, bantering with the nurses and discussing the Constitution with the young doctor who came to see him. No one seemed to know what to do.

Then the chief nurse of the psychiatry unit came in to give him a complete evaluation. When she finished, she took me into the hall and said that he seemed just to be suffering from some of the effects of LBD and that we needed to check his medications. I asked if they could do it at the hospital, and she said, "Honey, you call that memory care facility and tell them to get their doctor over there and that you are bringing Don back. This man is not psychotic."

Then another fortuitous thing happened. The VA called and said that they had a new psychiatrist in our district, and she would like to talk to us and get acquainted with Don. I called her back immediately and explained the situation. We scheduled a Zoom meeting at the memory care unit for the next day. Greg and I took Don back to his room and stayed with him until he was asleep. We asked the nurses to only give him Tylenol for his back pain until after the doctors had evaluated the meds.

The following day Greg and I arrived at the Zoom meeting in business suits with clipboards and handouts. The director of the facility, the director of the memory care unit, Don, my son, and I all sat at a long table and connected with the VA psychiatrist. I had emailed her Don's complete medical history, so she was well briefed. The VA doctor started the meeting by talking to Don and asking him if he had any concerns. She listened carefully and respectfully to his somewhat disjointed comments and then asked me to summarize what had been happening.

I had made a timeline that listed all of Don's medications and the concerns we had about placing Don in a psychiatric ward. I gave everyone a copy. Again, the doctor listened carefully to me and then directed questions to the facility directors.

After hearing from all sides, she said that it seemed that Don had LBD and was suffering from delusions and hallucinations. She asked the memory care director to have their doctor contact her as she wanted some of his medications changed immediately. She explained that the drug they had been giving Don to reduce anxiety was usually well tolerated by dementia patients but not those with LBD. And the VA psychiatrist was correct. Don never had another major psychotic episode!

I sold our house, but Brad's place was unavailable, so I moved into a "respite" room in the assisted living place where Don's memory care facility was. I had a bed, two card tables, a chair, several boxes, and a dog. My main goal was to be near Don during the first few weeks and learn how the memory care unit worked. During my thirty-plus-some years of teaching, I found that it is the informal management system that you need to tap into. Usually, the most influential person in the school is not the principal but the custodian! So, I made sure that I became friends with the maintenance guy, the receptionist, the custodian, the cook, and all the aides and nurses!

I brought snacks, remembered birthdays and holidays, wrote notes for the "You've been noticed board," and thanked everyone! It was the custodian who inspected the trash cans in Don's room to make sure that Don hadn't thrown away his dental plate and who found his TV remote. The nighttime aide took me aside and suggested I buy colored sheets for Don's bed. She told me that, in her experience, dementia patients weren't as likely to pull off the sheets if they were brightly colored.

The staff would call me and tell me when the hair salon was open so I could make an appointment to get Don's hair cut or let me know that he was out of incontinence briefs. I also tried to introduce Don to the staff. I wanted them to see him as a person, not just someone they had to clean up and feed. They were especially impressed with the picture of Don and his partner in the local "Dancing with the Stars" event and all his medals. Gradually, Don relaxed and started interacting with both residents and aids.

Often conversations between residents were both amusing and heartbreaking. I came in one day and found Don and a lady talking away, both laughing and smiling. When I sat down and listened, I realized that the lady thought Don was her father, and Don thought she was an old schoolmate.

Most people in the memory care unit were females with Alzheimer's. Because of the COVID restrictions, they no longer had many visitors or volunteers. All the activities listed on the colorful website no longer existed. There was no "customized musical playlist," no fun exercise sessions, and no volunteers to engage the residents. The dementia patients were left alone except for meals and medications. Most just sat in their wheelchairs and walkers and twisted their hands.

Don loves music, so I learned how to operate the small TV in the common area with the music channel. Then we could have sing-a-longs and dance parties. Amazingly, many patients who barely talked could sing, and some still danced. I named one petite little woman "The Dancing Queen" because she really had the moves – I could never shimmy like that.

I also brought in simple crafts such as pasting colored hearts on paper wreaths for Valentine's Day, making Madi Gras masks, and Christmas snowmen. Don never participated in these activities because his coordination was poor, but he loved watching. I was also able to have Recon recognized as a therapy dog. I brought him in several times a week. He always made a beeline for Don but then was glad to be petted by the other residents. They all loved throwing a stuffed toy, watching Recon retrieve it, and sitting for his treat. Using his walker, Don would walk around the grounds with me, identifying birds and flowers and just watching the clouds.

Things smoothed out, and as the COVID pandemic slowed, we had a cookout, special ice cream days, and holiday treats. Our family would come with pizza or donuts when visitors were allowed back. Some friends brought their dogs or pictures of Don in happier days. We could go for long drives and stop for picnics.

One of my special memories is of the Veteran's Day cookout. All veterans in his assisted living facility and memory care were recognized in a special program, and the Hospice Chaplin gave a short talk. They played the anthems for each branch of our military services, and I helped Don stand for the Marine Corps hymn. Later that evening, we had a cookout with a disc jockey. Several family members and a few residents were dancing to rock and roll songs, and suddenly Don jumped up to join them. He was moving and grooving! I, and every aide there, dashed over to form a circle around Don so that he couldn't fall. He looked so happy – ten ladies dancing and clapping with him! I asked the disc jockey to play some slow dance music, and we danced until dark. It was the last time I ever danced with him.

Several people visiting Don had a difficult time communicating with him. They were very uncomfortable, and many just never came back. However, our grandchildren were wonderful. Whenever the family arrived, they brought snacks and drinks. Eating made it more festive and relaxed. Often Don couldn't follow the conversation so he would interrupt with a completely irrelevant comment. "On the farm, I had a horse named Joko." The grandkids would turn their attention to Don and ask questions. "Did you ride a lot?"

They seemed able to relate to him as he was. All of them made Don feel included and loved. One afternoon our youngest grandson, Chris, was home from college. He had come to visit, and when he saw the grand piano at the main entrance, he asked Don if he would like to listen to some music. Don was always ready to listen to music, so Chris pulled out a vintage songbook and played old favorites. Soon we had an audience enjoying" Amazing Grace" and "In the Good Old Summertime."

Don smiled and tried to sing along. When I pushed him back to the memory care unit, he smiled back at me. "That was a happy place."

Don still asked every day, "Can we go home now?" His main problems, besides progressive dementia, were his painful back, falling, constipation, and boredom. I couldn't always be there all the time, and the aides didn't have much time to interact with the patients.

He became increasingly delusional, often thinking he was back on the farm or in the Marine Corps. I had to keep explaining to him that the residents were not in the Marine Corps and didn't have to obey his orders. One day when I visited, he insisted that we "inspect" the security at the facility. I pushed him all around the building, stopping at doors and entranceways so he could check them out. He was not impressed, and when we returned to the memory care unit, he suddenly stood up and bellowed, "OK, troops. Listen up. I'm sick and tired of the sloppy security and maintenance in this place." Then he gave a loud, somewhat incoherent yet inspirational speech about how everyone needed to work together and do their part. The aides and the other patients just listened and didn't seem to know how to react. Then one sweet, white-haired lady started clapping, "Amen! Good speech!" she called.

My relationship with the management of the facility was more confrontational. I often stopped by to "make suggestions" about more activities for the residents or ask why they could not maintain the appropriate staff-to-resident ratio. I would request that the cook be reminded that Don had to have his food cut into small bites or that he needed to have his incontinence briefs changed every two to three hours. I wrote letters requesting that his meds be crushed and given to him with applesauce or that they monitor his constipation problems more carefully. I couldn't help but worry about patients who didn't have someone visiting them every day and overseeing their care. Most of the aids were terrific, providing loving care for $15 an hour, but some seemed to spend most of the day on their phones!

I often felt that management was more concerned with filling their rooms than providing excellent service. One evening I came in and found only two aides on duty. I helped feed the residents and then had to call Brad to help me get Don in bed. The two female aides couldn't move him, and only one nurse and an aide were in the assisted living area. The next day, I visited the director and told her that having so few caregivers on duty genuinely concerned me. I asked what would happen if they had a fire. How could two aides help 22 dementia patients evacuate the building? She assured me that the caregivers knew what to do.

The next day I came in and found five aides and the director of the memory care unit busy getting patients out of their rooms and seated in the common area. One caregiver was sitting at a table cutting out green squares. When I asked what was happening, she replied that they would have a fire drill that afternoon, and she would tape the squares to each door as each resident left the building. Sure enough, the alarm went off at the appointed time, and six staff members and three visitors tried to herd the residents out the door into the parking lot. It was a fiasco. There was no ramp at the back parking lot, so little ladies in walkers couldn't get off the curb. One woman kept fighting to go back inside and get her coat. Residents who could walk were pushing wheelchairs for other residents. Once outside, the aides couldn't keep the patients confined to one area. The patients would wander off toward the street or stumble into the grass. No one seemed to know what to do. It was scary! Again. I issued a formal complaint.

Then we had the bedbugs. I would never have known about the infestation of bed bugs if a "porch buddy" – a family member who often met with his dad while I had Don on the porch– hadn't told me. All the family members who used the porch shared snacks and traded information. This gentleman was an exterminator by trade and told the manager that he had found bed bugs in his father's room. The manager insisted that they did not have bugs. The family member had to call corporate headquarters and demand they send out an inspector. Family members were not contacted. Since I had been warned, I carefully inspected Don's room each day and found several tiny bugs under his chest of drawers. I took some pictures and then sprayed the area.

Then I took the pictures to the director and told her where I had found them. She condescendingly explained that I was wrong, that the photographs were of common little beetles. As I was walking out fuming, I saw a woman in a uniform with" Exterminators" printed on it. Racing after her, I showed her my pictures. She agreed that they were bedbugs and marched back into the office. The next day, the director emailed all family members explaining that "someone" had brought bed bugs into the facility but that they would have the place sanitized immediately. Sure enough, the exterminators came and carefully cleaned each room. My porch buddy suggested that I take home all of Don's clothes and wash them with hot water. I brought my own sanitizers and bug spray after that.

I had a professor at grad school who told us that every ridiculous regulation we had in public schools was because someone did something stupid. And the legislators, instead of just chastising that person, created a new law that pertained to everyone. Memory care units were no different. One of the rules that caused Don many problems was the one that stated that memory care caregivers could not restrain patients. The regulations were issued when inspectors found some facilities strapping patients into beds at night so they would not have to check on them every two hours. But the law covered far more than bed straps!

At home, Don had slept in a hospital bed with a bed rail that I could raise at night. It kept him from falling out of bed during a dream and allowed him to pull himself upright. After we moved that bed into Don's room at the memory care unit, I came in one morning and found the rails gone. I found an aide who told me the director said they had to be removed. Instead, they placed a bed pad on the floor so if Don rolled out of bed; it would cushion his fall! So now Don could (and did) easily roll out. It was challenging for him to pull himself upright. When he tried to step on the floor, he was on a rubbery, unstable surface, so his falls increased. I asked Greg to find out precisely what the state law required. I researched online and talked to friends with medical backgrounds. It was true. Assisted living, memory care units and nursing homes cannot use any restraining device! That meant when Don started using a wheelchair, we could not buckle him in. So, he would bend down to pick up his fork and tumble forward onto the floor or decide to "exercise" and stagger down the hall.

One evening an aide called me and said that Don had fallen and gashed his head, and it was bleeding profusely. She said she thought he needed to go to the ER for stitches. I went over and found Don sitting in his wheelchair with a blood-soaked towel taped over his forehead. I asked the aide what happened, and she said that they were getting everyone ready for bed, and Don was sitting in this wheelchair contentedly watching a rerun of The Lone Ranger. She entered another resident's room and later heard a loud thump and yell. Don was lying on the floor at the end of the hallway with blood all over him and the corner of the hall table. She said that when she asked him what happened, Don replied, "I was taking off down the runway, and this table jumped out in front of me."

The aide said she couldn't help but laugh and told him, "Dude, you forgot your parachute!"

I took Don to the emergency room four times in one year for stitches. He fell an average of once a week and always seemed to have a new bruise or bump when I visited him. I asked the aides not to close his door at night so they could glance in and see if he was still in bed! I had made friends with many residents, and they watched him also. When Don tried to push himself out of the chair, a chorus of dear ladies would yell, "Don! Sit down!"

Urinary infections continued to be a problem. During one of the times, I took Don into the ER for stitches, they discovered he was running a temperature. I told them he had a history of urinary infections, and when they ran the test, it came back positive. Since his head wound was still seeping blood and his temperature was elevated, they decided to keep him overnight. I gave them the list of prescribed medications and explained that he had LBD. I asked them to put a note on his chart not to provide him with any painkillers or sedatives, such as morphine, because it would cause him to become manic.

When Don went to sleep, I left to go home, walk the dog, and get some sleep. I received a call the following morning at 7:00. "Please come in at once. We have to restrain your husband." When I arrived at his room, Don was lying on the bed with wrist restraints, yelling and twisting. One tall, attractive nurse in pink scrubs had him by the ankles lifting his legs off the bed so another lady could clean his bottom. When they saw me, they looked worried, afraid I would be upset. I just laughed and said, "You're doing great, Wonder Woman!"

I hugged Don and teasingly told him, "Just relax, Babe. You now have three beautiful women fussing over you." But it wasn't a laughing matter. Someone had given Don morphine overnight, and he woke up demanding that he had to get up and leave! Don was fighting the nurses and aids, threw his breakfast across the room, and kept trying to throw himself out of bed. I stayed with him all day, trying to keep him calm by singing, telling stories, and rubbing his back, until he finally fell asleep. Don was in the hospital for nine days while they tried to adjust his meds, control his urinary infection, and do therapy for his back.

The only good thing from the entire episode was that one of the doctors took me aside and said, "Look, if you were my mom, I would recommend that you put Mr. Don in hospice care." I was aghast. Hospice was for people who were dying! He went on to explain that hospice care would provide:

- A weekly nursing visit.
- A supervising doctor.
- An aide came in once a week to do things like trim his nails and clean his dental plates.
- A social worker would visit him weekly to talk and ensure he was doing well.
- A chaplain.

They would also ensure that his medications were appropriate, and that Medicare paid for them. I signed up!

Don became more and more frail. He wouldn't wear his glasses or his dental plates. His hearing aides had been destroyed in the laundry, and Don hated the hearing contraption I would bring in. He had started to whisper, so it was difficult to hear him. Low blood pressure often caused him to become very dizzy, and once, he even lost consciousness. Tremors in his hands made eating difficult, and now someone had to feed him his meals. He had lost fifty pounds and weighed only 115. My handsome husband looked like a withered old man. But still, when I came in, he would hold out his arms and hug me. He hadn't forgotten.

One day I had just gotten out of the shower, and the memory care director called. "Teddie, I think you need to come in. I believe Don is transitioning."

"What?" I had visions of Don changing into a butterfly or floating off into the clouds.

She explained that he started choking during lunch, and his breathing was shallow.

I interrupted, "Are you trying to tell me that Don is dying?"

"Well, yes!"

I left at once with wet hair and the nearest clothes I could throw on. When I arrived, an aide was sitting with Don by his bed. Don looked grey and tired. He would take a deep breath and then let it out in a long "whoosh." He had a temperature of 103, and his heartbeat was erratic.

I asked them to call a hospice nurse. Then I sat on the bed so I could hold his hand. It was cold. I had read that even when a person seems unaware, they could often hear you. So, I started talking to him: telling him a funny story about Recon and the little girls' next store. I reminded him that our grandson was coming home from college this week and would come to visit. It was calm, soothing chatter.

The hospice nurse came and said that he did have signs of someone entering the "transitional" stage before the "active" stage of dying. She cautioned me that he might die or get better that day. She prescribed something for his fever and ordered some juice for me to spoon into his mouth carefully. Then everyone went back to their duties, and I sat there and watched him. He started sitting up, gasping, and throwing himself back on his pillow. I panicked and texted the boys. Greg and Brad, who live in Georgia, drove to the facility. Dave, who was in Arkansas, requested that we keep him posted; he would come if we needed him. Then we all three sat there and watched Don. We talked in hushed whispers, me stroking Don's hand and wondering, "Now what?"

Finally, I said, "Well, this is like an Irish wake, except we don't have a fiddle player. Why don't you guys get us some food, and I'll stay? There's nothing you can do to make him better."

They reluctantly agreed, and then I said goodbye to Don. I thought this was the end, and I wanted him to know how much I loved him. Don calmly slept when the boys returned with steak sandwiches and iced tea. We ate and had a frank discussion about cremation, funerals, and memorial services. After the night nurse came and checked Don out, we left and returned to Brad's house. I was now living with my middle son near the memory care unit. Exhausted, we all went to bed.

Greg had to return to Atlanta for a court hearing, so he stopped by memory care early the following day. He called me and said, "I just left Dad eating blueberry pancakes and flirting with the hospice nurse."

That same nurse told me that Don would probably go through several episodes like that before he died. I texted the boys and apologized for panicking!

Don was only in a memory care facility for a year. It felt like a lifetime. My life was complexly centered around visiting him, shopping for him, arranging visits with friends and families, and meeting with the memory care and hospice staff.

In the last few months, Don seemed to enjoy the friends we had made, taking long drives and walks, singing songs, and watching old movies. His condition continued declining, but we all thought he could stay there for several more years. One of the hospice nurses told me that the one predictable thing about LBD was that it was not predictable. So true.

At the end of April 2022, I arrived at the three o'clock shift change one afternoon. Don was not sitting in the common area, and his door was closed. I looked around and didn't see any staff I recognized. I entered Don's room and found him gasping and writhing on his bed. I touched his head, and it was burning up. He seemed unconscious and didn't respond when I spoke to him. I dashed out to the nursing station and explained the situation. I asked if they call hospice and the facility nurses. I returned, applied cool towels to Don's head, and tried to get him to sip some water. He was moaning and shaking. I felt so blasted helpless! The facility nurse arrived first and ordered some aspirin crushed in applesauce. There was no mention of his being ill on his chart, so we had no idea how long he had been like this. I decided to call 911 and get an ambulance. Don was being secured to the stretcher when the hospice nurse arrived. She explained that as I had signed him into hospice care, Medicare would not cover his emergency transportation or hospital care. I had run into this situation before, so I asked that she take him off hospice care while he was in the hospital.

Everyone who cares for a LO with LBD faces the same ethical question. When do we stop treating life-threatening situations and just let them die? I had agreed that Don should only receive palliative care when I signed on to the hospice program. But I couldn't stand seeing him in so much pain, so I asked him to be removed from hospice care. We checked in at the nearest hospital, and they ran tests to discover what was causing his high fever and pain. They came back positive for a urinary infection and bronchitis. Also, he couldn't seem to urinate. The on-call urologist tried to place a catheter and told me that the scar tissue in Don's urinary tract was completely blocking the opening.

Don was now crying and moaning, clutching his stomach and rocking back and forth. I asked the doctor for options. "You can try a surgical dilation and then use a catheter bag, or we can cut a hole in his stomach and insert a suprapubic catheter directly into the bladder. "

I knew we could also do nothing, and Don would die in terrible pain. The last time he had a surgical dilation, he had an adverse reaction to the anesthesia and the painkillers used afterward. Also, the last time Don had that procedure, he kept pulling the catheter out and spilling urine all over the bed. The doctor assured me that inserting a suprapubic catheter only required medication to numb the region being cut, and he wouldn't be in much pain afterward. I chose the suprapubic catheter. But then, the urologist said the procedure couldn't be done at this hospital. Don would have to be moved to another hospital twenty minutes away!

When we arrived, it was 2:00 am. The ambulance drove right into the emergency entrance. I parked and ran in, but there was no sign of Don. The young man at the ER desk said that it was too late for me to go inside the hospital and that I should return in the morning. I tried to explain what had happened, and he called the surgical ward. No one answered. He finally contacted a nurse who said the urology team was doing the procedure. I sat in the cold, nearly empty waiting room for an hour, and finally, the surgeon called me. "He's fine and is asleep. Go home, and I'll call you in the morning."

It was dark and rainy, and my GPS took me off the main route and down little twisty country roads. I was exhausted and shaking by the time I reached the house. I collapsed on the bed and lay there, my mind skittering back and forth. Should I call the boys? Was it too early to contact the memory care unit and explain what happened? I needed to make sure the emergency bag had a change of clothes. Did I do the right thing?

I texted my family the following morning and told them what had happened. I dropped Recon by a friend's house, grabbed a Starbucks, and drove to the hospital. I decided to wait and contact the memory care facility after I had spoken to the doctor. Don was still asleep when I arrived, but the nurse told me he had slept all night and his temperature was almost normal. He was urinating and didn't seem to be in any real pain. I sat down near Don's bed and held his hand, telling him I was there and he would be fine. He probably couldn't hear me, but it made me feel better. Then I called the memory care unit and told an aide to please get in touch with hospice care and the memory care director and tell them what had happened. I said I wasn't sure when Don would return to the facility. I had just relaxed and closed my eyes when my phone rang. It was the director of the memory care unit. She told me federal law didn't allow them to do skilled nursing. Cleaning and changing a suprapubic catheter were considered skilled nursing, so Don would have to leave the memory care unit. "What?"

"Yes, you have a week to remove everything from his room."

"But where can I take him? What if I can't find an opening?"

"The hospital has to care for him until you find a place. Good luck." The last chapter of Don's story had started.

Things that I Learned.

1. I mentioned this in the last chapter, but it bears repeating! Read all the rules and regs in the memory care handbook. I knew memory care units couldn't do skilled nursing, but I wasn't sure what constituted "skilled nursing." Don had an intermittent catheter once a week, so I performed that for him. When he was placed in hospice care, their nurse did it. I assumed the hospice nurse could also care for the suprapubic catheter. The memory care where Don was placed emphatically stated that he had to leave. Over a year later, I was talking to a friend who told me the same thing had happened to her. She called her husband's urologist, and he said that a caregiver could change the catheter bag. The suprapubic catheter had to be changed every six weeks, but that could be done by taking her husband to the urologist or hiring a registered nurse. So,

don't assume you have to place your LO in a nursing home if this happens. Check with your urologist.

Also, a regulation for memory care placement in Georgia stipulates that a patient must be mobile enough to move without assistance in an emergency. Don now needed help to move his wheelchair more than a few feet.

2. Even if your LO is in a care facility, have an emergency bag in your car. Have a copy of his current meds and medical records. Be sure you have a change of clothes, some incontinence briefs, sanitary wipes, gloves, and towels. You'll be ready if you must take your LO to the hospital. Don't forget an extra charger and a cord for your phone.

When your LO is still in a memory care unit, be sure you label everything. Not only does your LO leave his possessions all over the facility, but aides also often get clothes mixed up in the wash, and other residents wander into the unlocked rooms and pick up things that catch their attention. We found Don's picture of Recon in another resident's room and his TV remote in a potted plant! Residents were constantly arguing about who had whose walker. I bought Don a bright red one, and we decorated it with USMC stickers and red and gold ribbons!

Memory care facilities usually bathe a resident once a week. The website and brochure said aides would also help with tooth brushing and cleaning fingernails and toenails. I found that this often did not happen. When hospice care takes over, they are responsible for personal hygiene. However, aides are not allowed to cut fingernails and toenails. So, you can either hire a podiatrist to come in and do that or do it yourself. Don enjoyed listening to music while I gave him manicures and pedicures!

Our facility also promised that a hair salon on the premises would provide haircuts, beard trims, and shaves. However, with COVID, that service was canceled. I bought clippers and shaved Don's beard and cut his hair. Fortunately, he was no longer vain about his looks!

Once patients are enrolled in hospice care, Medicare pays for sanitation and hygiene supplies, medical equipment, sanitary wipes, incontinence briefs, and flushable wipes. They prescribe, order, and oversee medications paid for by Medicare and the patient's insurance. When the nurse realized I was interested in what Don was taking, she called me whenever they thought a change was needed. The hospice care team was a real blessing.

Earlier, I said I didn't feel I benefited from therapy, but I was blessed with an incredible support group. If you need to vent or have someone to talk to, you can always ask to speak to the hospice social worker or look for a caregivers' support group at your local hospital or senior citizen's council. Churches sometimes offer support groups. The LBD Association website also offers an online Facebook group. These groups can provide helpful hints on how to cope with life as an LBD caregiver. However, check with your LO's doctors before you change medications or treatments.

Even the very best facilities have problems. Remember, you are paying for your LO's care. Don't be afraid to speak up and ask for what you need. Keep copies of all correspondence just in case you need to contact the corporate office. I was always careful to be polite and not assign blame. I wanted to solve problems, not cause them! Praise staff and management whenever you can. The memory care facility had a "Caught Doing an

Excellent Job" bulletin board. I posted a comment every week thanking someone!

We all suffer feelings of guilt and inadequacy when we finally decide to place our LOs in a care facility. We feel we have failed, weren't good enough, or didn't try hard enough. But we are only human, and I was often so tired and stressed that I would forget to give Don his prune juice or charge his hearing aids. On bad days, I would lose my temper and walk away from my husband. Aides stay up all night and check on patients every two hours in a facility. If needed, the nurse can give them pain medication at 3:00 am.

There are people who clean their rooms, wash their clothes, help them bathe, and provide meals. You can become a loving friend or family member who provides oversight, entertainment, activities, and love.

Winter Leaves

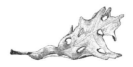

His mind, extinguished
His body, deceased
His spirit soars forever

When winter comes and the leaves turn brown, shrivel and eventually drop to the ground, we can still find pleasure in enjoying the snow or the festive preparations for winter holidays. But when your loved one reaches the last stage of Lewy Body Dementia, it is hard to find any solace.

It's hard to describe those eleven days in the hospital when my sons and I searched for a nursing home for Don. He seemed to have recovered from pneumonia, the urinary infection, and the supra pubic catheter procedure. But he was alternately passive and depressed or agitated and aggressive. I was there every day from nine in the morning until dinner. The doctor didn't want him to get out of bed, so I was constantly trying to find ways to entertain him when he was awake. One day my sister came to visit and we spent two hours looking up songs on our phones and singing them to Don. It broke my heart when he would try to sing along and couldn't remember the words. We were trying to harmonize to "You are my Sunshine" when one of the nurses walked in. "Are y'all practicing for American Idol?", she joked. Even Don laughed.

The boys and I spent hours on the computer looking up the ratings of local nursing homes and then calling to try and find an opening. Every place seemed to be filled. Our search expanded until we were looking at facilities over an hour away. Admission offices explained that while they had empty beds, they couldn't get enough staff to take care of their patients. We were close to panic.

Our standards had dropped from looking at outstanding ratings to average. With monthly prices ranging from $7500 to $9000, we even considered home care. But we knew that we wouldn't be able to find home nursing care either! We finally found a nursing home forty minutes away from my son's house with an average rating that was willing to take Don.

Greg and I went to see it and were delighted with the location. It was on several acres with trees, open fields, and flowers out front. The receptionist and the admissions director were both friendly and cheerful. However, the facility was slightly run-down, with depressingly dull walls and dirty windows. A small courtyard had a tree and some above ground vegetable planters, but the little pond had been drained and the flowers were in desperate need of watering and weeding.

Several residents in wheelchairs were watching a big TV in the common area and there were more clustered around the central nurses' station. Most rooms we passed were double occupancy and many had bedridden patients. A small dining area was currently closed because of the COVID pandemic, so patients had to eat in their rooms. Having no choice, I filled out the paperwork and paid the $7250.00 admission fee. I could not sleep that night. I had always told myself that I would never put Don in a nursing home, and now we were moving him in the next day.

I tried to suppress my anxiety and concerns, by gathering up what few personal items we could bring to his room. Brad's garage was filled with the things we had removed from the memory care facility, so I carefully picked out what we needed. The nursing home provided a hospital bed, linens, a small bedside table, tiny closet and a built-in counter with some drawers. Don's roommate already had a TV, so there was no room for another one. We brought pictures of the family, Recon, and Don's airplane plus a few clothes and toiletries. I kept a list of things I needed to do wash the dirty windows, bring in comfortable pillows, hand wipes, sippy cup for liquids, tissue, room deodorant, etc. We put a bird feeder outside his window and cleaned the area thoroughly. It was still very cramped, depressing, and sad.

Don was transported from the hospital by ambulance and brought into his room on a stretcher. The room was so small that Greg and I waited in the hall while the orderlies got him comfortable. There was only one chair in the room, so I had brought a small folding chair. We pulled the white curtain between the two beds and sat down. Don was awake and smiling, relieved to see us both. We brought snacks and a cozy blanket from the house, and just chatted until he fell asleep. He never once asked where he was or what had happened. Thankfully, he didn't seem to be frightened or upset.

And so the process started all over again. I brought brownies for the staff and wrote official letters to the management. The nursing home had a "circle meeting" for every patient every two months. Our first meeting went well. I met the head nurse, the chef, the new hospice team, and the social worker. Everyone was helpful and positive. I had brought a summary of Don's medical records and my requests for his care. They agreed to cut his food into small pieces and monitor his constipation. Now, he was still bedridden, but they assured me that they would get Don a Geri chair so I could roll him around the facility. I soon found out that the decisions made in the "circle" were not necessarily put into practice!

I would come in and find Don trying to get out of bed, with a dirty shirt and pieces of food all over the floor. It took two weeks to get the movable Geri chair and Don was going stir crazy. His roommate had the TV on all day, and I often brought "Mr Joe" brownies to sweeten my request to turn it off while I was there. Many of the aides were competent and helpful, but a sizable group just sat in the break room and looked at their phones.

One day I came in to find Don complaining of pain in his stomach. I asked the nurse if he had a bowel movement that day and she just looked at me like I was crazy. I asked to see his medical notes and she said they were in the head nurse's office. I asked to see the head nurse and was told she was out of the building. I went back to Don's room, and he was clutching his stomach and moaning. I rolled him over on his stomach and could see impacted feces. I went back to the nurse and told her that he had an impacted bowel. She stopped putting pills into little cups and asked "What do you want me to do? Call an ambulance?"

The last thing I wanted was the trauma of another hospital stay. I blurted out," No! I want you to help me." She replied that she was busy and would call an aide. When no caregiver came, I put on gloves and lubricant and removed the impacted material. Don immediately had a large bowel movement. After I cleaned everything up, he went right to sleep. I was so angry I was shaking. I marched up to the nurses' station and saw the head nurse was back. I went into her office and told her what had happened. She listened calmly and said "We'll increase his fiber. It will be OK."

In the six months Don was in the nursing home there were numerous crises. We had a huge water leak in the ceiling by his room, two urinary infections, a broken wheelchair that took two weeks to get repaired, and numerous incidents of just basic neglect. He would get so bored that he would try to get out of bed, and I often found him caught in the guard rails or hanging over the side of the bed. Sometimes there were only two aides and a nurse there in the evening with forty patients. What would happen if there was an emergency? It was so frustrating because there was no other place else to take him!

Fortunately, Don was in his own little world. I would come in and he would ask me to help him plan the annual airshow or suggest we could go outside and ride horses. One day I came in and he spent the entire time I was there explaining how the retired officer's club was going to have a turkey shoot in the nursing home's little courtyard. He asked me to take notes for the next board meeting. Little things became big victories. I was able to get the aids to use a lift to move him from the bed into a wheelchair. Then I could take him outside and walk around the grounds. The COVID restrictions were lifted, and I would come in and help with country music day or the ice cream sundae social. As I could move him around, I introduced him to the custodian, the cook and the other patients. I had an old CD player and often would have several patients in wheelchairs grouped around Don while we played Patsy Cline or Top Hits of the Sixties. As Don's tremors increased, I came in every day at about 3:30 and stayed until supper so I could feed him.

Unlike the residents of the memory care unit, many of the patients in the nursing home had serious physical ailments but were still mentally sharp. There was a group of ladies that I saw every day and we became good friends. I called them Don's Guardian Angels because they helped me look after him. I'd walk in and one would scoot her chair over to tell me that Don had really enjoyed his lunch in the cafeteria or that he had broken his sippy cup and needed a new one. Don was always trying to get out

of his wheelchair. The ladies would remind him to stay seated and then try to entertain him. I came in once and they were circled around him throwing a small pillow back and forth. One told me that he was really restless, so they were trying to distract him.
In return, I brought them magazines and flowers from the garden. Twice a week I would bring in doughnuts or chocolate chip cookies. I painted watercolor flowers in their favorite colors and hung them on their walls. They cheered me up and made Don feel at home.

Hospice care got Don a small wheelchair that he could scoot around with his feet. When he was feeling good, he would push himself up and down the halls under the watchful eyes of his "Guardian Angels". As he could not be strapped into the chair, he would often catch his foot and fall forward out of his chair. Fortunately, he weighed only 110 pounds and couldn't stand up, so he would usually just kind of slide on to the floor. The aides tried to keep him near the nurse's station so they could keep an eye on him.

My life centered around the nursing home. Get up and have breakfast, walk the dog, straighten the house, pay bills. Then get gas, snacks for Don and friends, perhaps shop for a new shirt or a clean pair of slippers for Don. It was a 45-minute drive to the nursing home and when I arrived, I usually cleaned him up, asked the aides to use the lift to get him in his chair and then I took him to the common area for a snack. If the weather was pretty, I took him outside and pushed him around the grounds. We'd look at the flowers and the clouds and I'd play music on my phone. I usually stayed until dinner so I could feed him and clean up the mess. Then I would push him to the common area, and we would join some of the other patients watching the big TV. Don couldn't really follow the show, but he enjoyed the chatter and the company. At about seven, I was able to get him into bed and the night nurse would give him his nighttime meds. Then I would go home and walk the dog.

On his 87th birthday, I brought in an ice cream cake, festive napkins and plates, balloons, and party hats. We went to the common area and set up the "party" on a small table. Everyone who passed was offered a piece of cake. We sang Happy Birthday, and I fed Don cake. Visitors, residents, and staff would pass and say, "Happy Birthday".

Don would smile and say, "Happy birthday to you too!"

Family and some loyal friends still came and visited occasionally. But as Don couldn't really communicate, the visits were more for me than him. I could certainly understand why people would not want to come. Usually there was at least one resident in a wheelchair right outside the front door just sitting in the sun. A few would be clustered in front of the big TV watching old sitcoms or westerns. The rest were either bedridden or sitting in their chairs beside their doors. One little lady constantly walked up and down the halls with a rag, "cleaning" the railings. Another sat in her bed moaning and calling out "Someone help me" over and over. Aides changed sheets and the duty nurse passed out pills. The place always smelled of urine and disinfectant.

After his birthday, Don started sleeping more and more. Often when I visited, he didn't open his eyes and just held my hand. He no longer seemed interested in eating. When I was there, I sat and talked about our lives together, told him about our sons and grandchildren. Music and singing seemed to soothe him, so I always brought CD's. Then the hospice nurse took me aside and said that he thought Don had entered the end stage.

I went home and immediately Googled "LBD End Stage". And then I made an appointment with the hospice social worker. The meeting went well. The young social worker was empathetic, but businesslike. I was numb. I felt I had told Don goodbye that night at the memory care facility when we were told he was "transitioning.' That evening I sat alone with him and told him how much he meant to me and to his family. I told him that he was a good, caring person and had contributed so much to our family, our country, our community, and friends. I told him that I would take good care of Recon and that I loved him very, very much. So now death was near, and I had already cried my tears.

The social worker told me exactly what I had read online. The main goal now was to keep Don comfortable; physically and emotionally. He could eat whatever he wanted and could swallow. He would be given medications to make sure he wasn't in pain and that he could breathe easier. She said that if we wished, the Chaplin would visit more frequently. I told her that we had made arrangements at a funeral home for Don to be cremated and gave her the name and number. It was all professional and somehow comforting. He had fought this awful condition so long and hard. We were both so very tired.

So, for the next week, I came in and stayed longer. I rubbed his skin with lotion and cleaned between his toes. I bought Dairy Queen ice cream and chocolate pudding. I played his favorite songs, held his hand and rubbed his back. His lady friends would stop me in the hall and ask for news. Some said that they went into his room during the day and talked to him. Greg and Brad came to visit, Dave and his wife, Mel called on Facetime, and we all just waited.

He became stiffer, rarely opened his eyes, and just stopped eating. Every time I came in, I would wet his lips and spoon tiny bits of water, until he turned his head away. It was late September, and the leaves were scarlet and gold, Marine Corps colors. I would sit by his bed and watch the clouds drift by. Two days before he died, he gripped my hand tight and whispered, "Teddie, I love you so darn much." I embraced him and told him I felt the same and reminded him that we always said that we would be together forever. It was the last time he spoke.

The next day I went in to find his bed gone. Don's roommate, who had become a friend, told me that they had moved him. I ran to find the nurse and they said that they had moved him to a private room on the far side of the building. No one else was in that wing. They had stationed an aide I had never met in a chair beside his door. She had orders to call the hospice office if there was any change in his condition. I went in and Don was lying in a dark, bare room with the shades drawn in the classic mummy pose – arms crossed over his heart. He looked like one of the stone effigies that you see in European cathedrals. I was truly shaken. I opened the shades and let sunlight in, covered him up and took his hand. I sat and watched him breathe in shaky little breaths. I couldn't talk without crying, so I just hummed. Greg arrived and I was so grateful not to be alone.

We just sat there and watched him and talked. Don barely seemed to breathe, but he didn't seem to be in any discomfort. We finally left and went home to call family. The nursing home called me the next morning as I was walking out the door. Don had just died.

It was surreal. I walked into the facility, and everyone looked solemn and sad. The dear ladies came up and patted my hand; hugging me and saying how sorry they were. The nursing home social worker met me and said that the funeral home had been called, but they knew I would like some time alone with Don. I walked in that dark, cold room and stared at Don. He looked like a mannequin, cold and lifeless. I didn't want to stay. Don was gone. There was only a husk left. Then I looked out the window and saw a hawk soaring over the green fields. I watched until it was out of sight.

"Vaya con Dios", I whispered. "I love you."

Things That I Learned

1.   As your LO becomes stiffer and has more tremors, it's hard to find comfortable clothes for them and it's always difficult to get a shirt or dress over their heads and arms. I purchased a very expensive shirt with a Velcro opening down the back and on the sleeves. It never seemed to fasten right! An aide suggested that I just buy women's yoga pants and shirts a size larger. No buttons, snaps or zippers, and they were comfortable and easy to get on and off. I shopped at discount stores; he no longer cared what brand they were. I also brought two pairs of slippers with Velcro straps, so I could take one pair home and wash them while he wore the other.

2.   You are your LO's advocate. I always kept copies of any correspondence with the management just in case I had to call the corporate office. Keep track of any doctor's appointment and remind the nursing home a few days ahead. Don had to have his catheter removed and cleaned every six weeks. I wrote the dates on my calendar and always reminded the head nurse a week ahead of time.

3.   Hospice is a true comfort and a wonderful resource. However, anytime you have to take your LO to the hospital, and they keep him over night, neither hospice nor Medicare will pay for the stay. You must contact your hospice office and take your LO off hospice care while they are in the hospital. That way Medicare will help with the bill. Also, once you are unable to transport your LO to the hospital or a doctor's appointment in your car, you have to call a special transport company for sick and disabled people. It cost me $600 to take Don back to the urologist for a follow up visit.

4. Experts believe that even when your LO does not seem to know that you are there, they still respond to sound and touch. Calm, happy voices, walks in the sunshine, loving hugs and holding hands provide reassurance and a sense of wellbeing. Patients often enjoy visits from their pets and special treats such as ice cream or pizza. Playing or singing their favorite music seems to soothe restless or agitated patients.

5. Some LBD patients are restless and agitated and will often "pick" at things. They will pluck at their sheets and try to throw the blanket off the bed. They will pull tissues out of the box and tear up paper cups. To keep their hands busy, some nursing homes have "fiddle" toys. These might be boards with items that can be manipulated, or rubber balls you can squeeze. Don seemed to enjoy stroking a small stuffed bear. Ask the aids and nurses for suggestions.

6. When your LO stops eating and drinking, most experts in dementia suggest that he not be given a feeding tube. They stress that the tube just causes the patient stress and discomfort. They suggest that you merely offer foods that your LO enjoys and can swallow – you don't have to follow a diet now. If he can suck, try Frosties or thin milk shakes. As the end grows near, just wet their lips with a cloth, or offer a small spoonful of liquid. Don't try to force them to eat or drink; they may choke or spit it out.

7. Try to finalize funeral arrangements early. It took me forever to write an obituary for Don. I sent copies to each of our sons, and they all had their own suggestions. Many LO's have already made their preferences known, so you can just follow their wishes. If they haven't, certainly be open to your family's ideas, but do what you feel your LO would want. We decided on a celebration of life instead of a funeral.

8.   Check with your lawyer and your banks as to what you should do when your LO dies. As a military wife, I had a long list of agencies I had to contact. I used every one of the ten official death certificates I ordered. Even if you are the only beneficiary, you may need to probate the will and get a letter of testamentary. I found that one of our financial institutions wouldn't send me a copy of Don's tax form until I sent them a copy of the letter of testamentary. Also, ask your bank how long you should keep your LO's name on your joint account. I found that I was receiving small checks from various companies and agencies many months after Don died. They were all addressed to his estate. As your power of attorney is no longer in effect when your LO dies, you can still deposit the checks in your joint account - if his name is still on the account!

The weeks right after your LO dies are very stressful. You still haven't processed their passing and you have to sign forms, handle the insurance, contact institutions. You need to make decisions about the funeral or memorial, contact extended family and close friends, and pay bills. Ask for help. Talk to your spiritual leader, a therapist, or a close friend. Try to find some time to just be by yourself and grieve. Don died at the end of September, and I took a long weekend to go to the beach in October. I told family that I didn't want to join the annual family Christmas celebration that year. I didn't feel I could be festive and merry.

Remember the good times and don't dwell on the things you couldn't change. You did the very best you could in a heartbreaking, stressful and physically demanding situation. Be kind to yourself. It's now a new chapter in your life.

Timeline

2015: Don suffered a compressed disk fracture, triggering a physical and cognitive decline.

2016: Don's health and cognitive/emotional condition continued to decline. My search for answers begins.

2017: We downsize to an over fifty community. Hallucinations and delusions begin.

2018: Don is diagnosed with "unspecified dementia" and loses his driver's license—caregiving tips on coping with symptoms of LBD.

2019: The COVID pandemic causes isolation, problems getting home health aides, and depression. Delusions, sundowning, and wandering become worse.

2020: Physical conditions such as falls, impacted bowels, incontinence, urinary infections, and urinary retention worsen. Parkinson- like symptoms such as tremors, balance, and speech problems increase. My back and a detached gluteus medias make it more difficult for me to care for Don.

2021: We move Don to a memory care unit and try to cope with the problems that it causes. He is placed in hospice care.

2022: Don is placed in a nursing home and enters the end stage of LBD.

Epilogue

Stages of Grief

- **Denial**
- **Anger**
- **Why Me?**
- **Depression**
- **Acceptance**

With dementia, the stages of grief happen when your LO is first diagnosed, and you realize there is no cure. Then it happens again when he dies.

First, there is the immediate stomach punch. He's gone! Then you have weeks or months dealing with the funeral, death certificates, the will, paperwork, and financial problems. But the day finally comes when you can take a deep breath and ask, "Now What?"

This was the first time I did not have a partner in sixty years. There was no one to help me plan the garden or the next vacation. No one to turn to when watching the news and ask, "Can you believe this?".

My family and friends are wonderful. But after a lovely evening out, I'll drive home alone and think, "Don would have loved that band." And I'll start to cry. Several of my friends have lost their husbands, and they all said to give it time, and things would get better. The ache would not go away, but it would soften.

So, I went to the beach and walked along the sand, looking for shells. I visited my family and reconnected with friends. I took a writing class and started doing watercolor painting again. I worked in my garden and joined the YMCA. And I started writing this book. First, to process what had happened to Don and me. But then to help others deal with LBD.

However, I am no longer young. When I think about volunteering with an organization, I am reminded that I have mobility issues and wonder if I could contribute anything. I find I don't have the energy to start a new project or take a long trip to South Africa. I have to assess what I want to do and if I can do it. The words of Janis Joplin's song, "Me and Bobby McGee," come to mind. "Freedom's just another word for nothing left to do."

But I trust life will be whole again. I will cherish the people in my life now but actively seek out new places, challenges, and friends. I am planning a cruise to the Caribbean and hope to do some events to raise money for research into LBD. I want to learn Tai Chi and join the arts council.

An elderly friend told me many years ago, "There will always be a new spring." I believe that. But I will always miss Don.

About the Author

Teddie Potter was a Marine Corps brat and then married a Marine. Some of her earliest memories are of packing up the car and heading off to a new home, new school, and new friends.

She married Lt. Donald Lohmeier in 1962 and they had three remarkable sons, Greg, Brad and David. Don was overseas or on deployment about half of his 24-year career, including two tours in Vietnam. However, the family enjoyed traveling and experiencing new places.

Teddie attended one year of college at the University of South Carolina, and then spent the next thirteen years taking courses whenever she could. She received her undergraduate degree in history from the University of North Carolina, her master's degree in learning disabilities from Columbia College in Georgia, her specialist degree in gifted education from Valdosta College and finally after ten different schools, her doctorate in educational leadership from the University of Georgia.

After retiring she and Don were active in community activities, traveled extensively and enjoyed spending time with their family. After Don developed Lewy Body Dementia, she took care of him at home for six years and then was his advocate and daily visitor when he had to be moved to a memory care facility and later, a nursing home.

Her hobbies are reading, travel, gardening and doing watercolors. Blessed with a loving, supportive family and friends, she's trying to honor Don's life by supporting research for Lewy Body Dementia.

One hundred percent of all profits from this book will be donated to the LBDA.

Made in the USA
Las Vegas, NV
05 September 2024

94821903R00059